A Dance in the Desert

Mindy Gibbins-Klein

Ecademy Press

A Dance in the Desert first published in 2001
2nd revised and updated edition published in 2004
This 3rd revised edition published in 2009 by;
Ecademy Press
6, Woodland Rise, Penryn, Cornwall, UK. TR10 8QD
info@ecademy-press.com
www.ecademy-press.com

Printed and Bound by; Lightning Source in the UK and USA
Set in Garamond by Charlotte Mouncey
Printed on acid-free paper from managed forests. This book is printed on demand, so no copies will be remaindered or pulped.

ISBN 978-1-905823-57-4

The right of Mindy Gibbins-Klein to be identified as the author of this work has been asserted in accordance with sections 77 and 78 of the Copyright Designs and Patents Act 1988.

A CIP catalogue record for this book is available from the British Library.

All rights reserved. No part of this work may be reproduced in any material form (including photocopying or storing in any medium by electronic means and whether or not transiently or incidentally to some other use of this publication) without the written permission of the copyright holder except in accordance with the provisions of the Copyright, Designs and Patents Act 1988. Applications for the Copyright holders written permission to reproduce any part of this publication should be addressed to the publishers.

Copyright © Mindy Gibbins-Klein 2001, 2004, 2009

*In memory of my father, a great writer and a great friend.
And in honor of my mother, a constant source of inspiration.*

Chapter 1

As she opened the curtains, Kate felt the hot Arizona sun and it seemed to burn through her skin and enter her bloodstream. All of a sudden, she felt a tremendous heat in her body, and an accompanying lethargy like a heavy blanket thrown across her legs. *Perfect pool weather,* she mused, thankful for the thousandth time that she had decided to move to Arizona. Kate opened the sliding glass door which led from the living room onto the terrace and stepped out in her bathrobe.

The shrieks and cries of the children in the pool were an appropriate background to Kate's thoughts of the upcoming week. With only a few days left to the summer, she felt as though she was falling down a long spiral into a black hole. And there was a strong gravitational pull sucking her down faster than she was willing to go. Of course, Kate looked forward to going back to the school, as she did each September, but it was in a vague, intellectual way, remembering the fact that she enjoyed teaching the students but not any of the emotions attached to the memory. *Strange,* she thought, *how a two month summer can seem like an eternity, but I feel as though I haven't done anything.* With the renewed resolve that comes to those who see the end approaching, she went into the house to make some coffee.

As Kate stirred the one level teaspoonful of sugar into her coffee, she was again plagued by a sense of loss, of the perfect summer being yanked out from under her, with nothing yet to replace it. She consoled herself with a promise to drive out to the Desert Botanical Gardens one day during the week, to see the multi-colored cactus flowers one last time and imprint the scene in her memory for a "rainy day". The expression made Kate smile, for in the three years she had been in Arizona, she had not seen an entire day of rain. The Arizona sky held out for weeks on end, then spat out a light shower or even downpour, but it never lasted more than a few hours. Kate liked to imagine the sun overpowering the clouds and bursting in to disperse them, refusing to be blocked any longer.

A loud knock on the glass door disturbed Kate's reverie. She could see Jackie looking at her watch and shifting her weight from one foot to the other impatiently.

"Come in, it's open!" Kate shouted, not wanting to get up from the kitchen table anyway. Jackie flung herself into the living room, and strode across towards Kate.

"Kate, you're unbelievable!" she cried. "You told me you would come by at nine o'clock so we could get good seats. I waited and waited. I thought maybe you overslept."

Kate jumped up from her chair. "Is today Wednesday already?" Jackie nodded, smiling at her friend. It was actually quite uncharacteristic of Kate to be so careless about schedules. A good sign; maybe two months of relaxing summer were finally having an effect. Too bad it was coming to an end.

"I'm so sorry," Kate was saying as she poured the remains of her coffee down the sink. "I really wanted to get some seats close to the front. We promised Sam and George we would be their good luck charms. What time is it, anyway?" she asked, looking at the kitchen clock as she said it. Only twenty minutes after nine. The tennis didn't actually start until ten o'clock, but the residents of Sunny Vista were sure to be getting to the courts early for the condominium championship they had been waiting all summer for.

Kate kept talking as she rushed around in her bedroom, getting dressed. "You know, I can't keep track of the days in the summer. They all seem to run together unless there is some special event, like today. But I guess my mind is too full of anxieties about going back to school." She couldn't hear any reply from Jackie, who had sat down to enjoy the air conditioning in the other room. Kate picked up her canvas bag and returned to the living room.

"Don't worry about it," Jackie said, getting up slowly as Kate entered the room. The air conditioning had cooled her substantially, and nothing seemed quite so urgent anymore. Jackie still had, as Kate did also, remnants of the East Coast mentality, a tendency to rush around frenetically, nervous about "getting everything done". But that was one of the reasons both women had moved to Arizona. First Kate had come out West, looking to forget the hustle and bustle of her New York existence, as well as the unpleasant memories of a failed marriage. Instantly cheered by the hot sun and more relaxed pace, she had encouraged Jackie to visit, and Jackie had taken a week's vacation and stayed with Kate. That was three years ago, or "three years and two months" as she was prone to say, counting the time passed in her new life as a child counts his age. And neither of the two had ever looked back.

"Ready?" asked Kate, opening the sliding door again. Jackie followed her outside and they walked in the sweltering mid-morning heat towards the tennis courts.

There were already about forty or fifty people in the stands, which were built to seat about half of the development's five hundred residents. The perennial problem was getting a seat in the shade, since the builders of Sunny Vista seemed to think it necessary that the development live up to its name, and there was a paucity of trees all over the grounds, but especially near the tennis courts.

Jackie pushed her way past a few people who were standing at the bottom of the stand, deciding where to sit. Kate followed closely behind, murmuring a quick apology as she sidled past the last of the group. Jackie had found two seats in the fifth row up from the courts. No shade, of course.

As Kate settled herself in the seat, she looked around for her friends Sam and George. Ever since she first moved into the development, she had enjoyed spending time with these two, and the proximity of their condo made it very conducive to get together often. Sam and George were both native Arizonians, had gone to college together in Tempe, and now shared a condo in Sunny Vista, close to their respective jobs in Scottsdale. Since the development was primarily geared for families, with its pools, playground, and day care center, the younger adults like Kate, Jackie, Sam, and George found each other a bit removed and out of touch. They usually sought out each other's company, feeling they could relate better in that environment. Kate was glad, however, when they mingled with other residents of the community, like today. It somehow made her life more real and gave her a chance to see children up close, helping her decide if that's what she wanted when she 'grew up'.

She spotted George almost immediately, with his shock of orange hair and white, freckled legs poking out of his tennis shorts. He was leaning against the equipment shed, stretching his calf muscles, which were undoubtedly still tight from the intensive practice over the past week. George looked up and Kate caught his eye. At once she smiled and pointed to her nose. George broke into a huge grin and nodded vigorously, signifying that he had remembered to put extra sunblock on.

Kate liked the way the foursome looked out for each other in this way. They were always there for each other, like the time Jackie's car wouldn't start and Sam drove her all the way into town, only to return and go in the other direction to go to his job. Kate felt lucky to have made close friends in this new place, after the sorrows she had endured in New York just before she moved.

Sam was hollering to Jackie and Kate across the court. "I hope you have your cameras ready because you are about to see history being made." He swung his racquet for emphasis and Kate laughed out loud. Sam came from a very long line of traditional Indian relatives, most of whom still lived on the reservation nearby. He had often told them about the clashes he had with the more conservative ("tight assed" was the way he put it) elders over issues like integrating with the surrounding community. Sam was about the most integrated person Kate knew, and his emotional outbursts were his way of rebelling against a too-strict upbringing. Jackie and Kate waved back at the guys just before they went into the Players Lounge to await the start of the championship.

The championship was an annual event at Sunny Vista, and, since so many residents took their tennis seriously (players and spectators alike), there was always a good turnout. George and Sam had both been finalists last year, and in the deciding set, Sam had beaten George 6-4. It had been great fun to watch the two friends struggle to the last, challenging each other to surpass any past performance and rise to the

Matt seemed to glide across the court as he beat the young player in game after game. When he had won the match, he jumped over the net quickly and gave his opponent a hearty handshake. He could be seen talking to him as they went into the Players Lounge, and Kate wondered briefly what he was saying.

But George was playing next and Jackie was taking photographs frantically. "Relax, Jack," laughed Kate. "You have the whole match to get the perfect shot." Jackie and George had always gotten along well, and when the foursome went out together, they often paired up and separated. Kate had an idea that it was to let her and Sam be alone together, but now, as she watched Jackie, she wasn't sure. George looked hot and tired, as he chased the balls his opponent was flinging in every direction. He seemed more relieved than upset when the match finally went to the Mad Ball-Flinger and he was free to cool down in the lounge.

Before long, Kate saw Sam coming towards the court, and he waved his racquet at them in victory. Apparently, his win in the back court had earned him a place in the finals. He broke into a jog as he approached the court and his longish black hair flying behind him reminded Kate of his Indian heritage. The profile as he rounded the bend confirmed this: the high cheekbones that gave him an air of pride and the thin lips set in determination. Sam took a long swig from his water bottle before entering the court for the final match.

Matt walked leisurely to his side and they stared at each other for a moment before commencing play. They were so evenly matched, these two, that sometimes it seemed like Kate was watching a mirror. Both Sam and Matt played at top speed and with as much energy as earlier in the day, despite the hours of challenging tennis each had already played. The points were few and far between, brilliant shots by one or the other that were too impossible to return. As they began the last game, with a tie score, the people in the stands seemed to hold their collective breath. They knew Sam as the development's resident tennis champ, but this newcomer was astounding. They could see from the way his body moved with grace and fluidity that he was also a pro.

One smash by Matt and the game, set and match were over. Kate looked anxiously at Sam, because she knew that he had looked forward to winning the championship for the third consecutive time. To her utter amazement, Sam threw his head back and laughed as he and Matt clapped each other on the back over and over, and shaking. They both stood arm in arm and bowed to the crowd, who were screaming with laughter. It was then that Kate noticed the flapping back portion of Matt's shorts, like a pair of Dr. Denton pajamas, obviously cut on purpose, as a cooling mechanism. The flap allowed everyone a clear view of Matt's backside, a large portion of it, anyway. He hurriedly redid some of the snaps before striding across to collect his trophy from the Association committee.

With the competition behind them, Sam and Matt led the remaining spectators to the pool area where they jumped into the largest pool with their clothes on. Before long, there were many residents in or around the pool area, some people bringing out food for dinner, bottles of wine, and blankets to sit on the grass. Kate and Jackie found a semi-secluded spot a bit away from the children where they could talk quietly. They were both conscious of the imminent end to a seemingly endless summer that had enhanced their friendship, allowing them to get to know each other better while exploring the deserts of Arizona. Not to mention that along with George and Sam, they had gained some sense of fulfillment as young adults making an exciting new start in life. Not for the first time, Kate contemplated how lucky she was to have found Sunny Vista and her neighbors.

"Here, catch!" Kate had to duck as a softball went whizzing by her head and rolled under a chaise longue by the pool. She whirled around to confront the ball-thrower who had almost hit her and saw the tall adolescent from the afternoon tennis match shrug his shoulders. "Sorry. Matt said you might want to throw a ball around with us. At least it didn't land in the water." He laughed with an embarrassed snort.

As she opened her mouth to retort, Matt called to her from a bit farther away. "You do play softball, don't you?" His smile was mischievous and unabashed. Kate let out a sigh, unable to stay angry at Matt or the boy.

"I'm not really in the mood," she explained, and turned around to talk to Jackie again. "I don't know what it is about him, Jack, but he infuriates me and intrigues me at the same time." Not sure whether this statement would open up a can of worms, Kate shifted uncomfortably in her seat. Jackie had been very supportive during the bad days with Mitch, inviting her to spend countless nights sleeping on her living room sofabed, listening over endless cups of coffee to Kate's lamentations of Mitch's alcoholic tantrums. Jackie had been the only one Kate had been willing to pour her heart out to as her world crashed down all around her, sending bits of her heart flying after the disintegrating fantasy. When it was time to let go and call it quits, it was Jackie who sat with her as she packed up her belongings, distracting her with funny stories about her work at the hospital.

This outpouring of emotion had acted like an anchor to Kate, who, ever since then had felt vulnerable and exposed. Although rationally she knew that she could trust Jackie like no one else, she still felt indebted to her from those days three and a half years earlier, like someone constantly at the heavy end of a see-saw. If only she could "lighten up" about it, as her therapist in New York used to say. God damn it, why had she discontinued therapy just when she was getting somewhere? She tried to shake off the feelings which invariably plagued her when she was with Jackie.

"I think he's fantastic," Jackie was saying. "Look at the way he's rounded those kids up for the game." They watched as Matt put his hands over one of the teenager's own hands around the bat to correct his stance.

"Maybe he'll improve the kid's average at the Lounge's plate glass windows." No one knew who had smashed the glass at the Players Lounge last month, but it was generally assumed it had been the development's own teenage residents, who were bored and restless and uncontrollable by their parents. Kate, from her work at the junior high schools, had developed a contempt for the disrespectful vandals, whose parents, it seemed, had never had time for them and now turned to the teachers to handle them. It was only the studious and attentive ones that made Kate's job worthwhile; she often complained to the other teachers at the school how the general standard was deteriorating.

Jackie did not see her point of view and called Kate intolerant and uncompromising, but then, she did not have to work with them on a regular basis. Not that Jackie's job as a nurse in Phoenix Hospital's maternity ward was easy, but at least her patients were usually appreciative by the end of their stays. This time, Jackie let Kate's comment pass, realizing that it was probably back-to-school anxiety that was bothering her friend. The evening passed in a long, luxurious stream, and culminated with a songfest at around midnight. In the three years that Kate had lived in Sunny Vista, she had never felt so much a part of the community. Her neighbors were just there, like the pool, or the flower beds, pleasant but not pertaining to anything personal. Now, as the variety of voices filled the summer air, she felt strangely content. The voice leading the group in familiar folk songs was strong and melodious. Kate could not see across the lawn, since the condominium lights had gone out at ten-thirty; lighted lawn torches flickered in earnest to set the mood. Jackie leaned over and tapped her shoulder. "Our Matt is just a multi-talented genius," she said breathily, and Kate's contentedness dropped in shards all around her.

So, it was Matt whose guitar and loud singing voice she could hear above all the others who were joining in. She should have known. What is *wrong* with him? she thought, sitting up straight. Why did he have to take over completely? The harmonious singing now seemed raucous and harsh.

Kate felt her own feelings of admiration, which apparently mirrored Jackie's, fighting against an unwillingness to let the stranger in, especially since he had changed the mood at Sunny Vista so abruptly and thoughtlessly. He even has his dog joining in, Kate realized, as the low tones of the golden retriever added their insult to her personal injury. She had no idea why she felt so threatened, and thinking about it was making her very tired. She said goodnight to Jackie, and left to go to bed, where she soon fell asleep against the muted singing of her neighbors.

Chapter 2

Dragging the heavy kayak in the dirt behind her, Kate brushed some strands of hair from her face with a sweaty palm and wondered briefly how she let herself be coerced into joining the group on this expedition. But the others were laughing and joking with no apparent difficulties, so Kate pulled harder on her kayak, catching up with George.

"Hey, lady," smiled George. His easy manner instantly relaxed Kate. It was remarkable how she could take this warm, affectionate person for granted sometimes, turning instead to Sam, with his passionate nature yet darker moods. Kate had slipped a few yards behind again in her daydreaming and she could see the backs of George's legs looking slightly pink already in the early morning sun.

"George, did you put any sunblock on the backs of your legs? I know, I know, 'Don't mother me'," Kate mimicked, not waiting for the inevitable moan from George. It was a standing joke between them that Kate could not stop mothering him, and George did not really mind at all. In fact, he quite liked the attention. "I'll put some extra on you before we go in the water," she concluded, feeling satisfied that she had done her job.

Once in the water, the group spread out; the current made it impossible for them to stay very close to one another, and the distance mingling with rushing water precluded any conversations of more than a few shouted syllables. Kate saw Jackie about two hundred yards ahead and she was happy that her friend was managing the kayak so well. She, meanwhile, was content to paddle slowly, letting the small boat do most of the work. She knew that this was one time she could not be in control without expending a lot of effort, so she gave it up and basked in the Arizona sun.

Matt approached her with a splash. "What did I tell you, isn't this the greatest?" He looked exactly as he had after the tennis matches and Kate caught her breath sharply.

"It *is* very relaxing," she agreed, wanting to say more, but feeling acutely self-conscious. She was grateful that Matt did not say anymore as they casually drifted downstream. Kate marvelled at the kayaks' synchronous cutting through the water, then noticed Matt finishing a series of knots in a rope that now tied the two boats together. She was instantly outraged. "What makes you think I can keep up with you? What makes you think I *want* to keep up with you?" she spluttered, while trying unsuccessfully with her wet fingers to undo the knots.

"It's easy. In fact, it's easier for two kayaks to travel together than apart. Less chance of one of them tipping over," he shrugged, lying back in his kayak. "And we will end up going slower than before," he assured her. Seeing that she was not convinced, he rolled his eyes. "Didn't you ever drive a big old American car?"

As the analogy sank in, Kate laughed and released her tight grip on Matt's kayak. "I suppose you're right," she agreed, and tried to relax back in her boat like Matt was.

"Besides," he continued, "I thought it would be a good chance for us to get to know each other better." When she looked at him, she saw an intense look as he stared directly at her. His natural smile belied any threatening implication, though Kate was still looking for some hidden meaning behind the words. "I actually feel kind of foolish," Matt confessed. "The kayaking is a blast, but it's not really a group activity. We probably won't see the others until we get to Paw Junction in about an hour."

"That's all right," countered Kate, "since we can't hear each other much over the water. And I'm not one for much talking anyway." Having said that, she suddenly felt ill at ease, as though Matt could see right through her bathing suit and shorts. *Not one for much talking, my foot,* argued her inner voice. *Within about two minutes, you'll be talking your head off about all kinds of nonsense, like you always do.* She never knew how to deal with this negative self-talk, the poisonous enemy of her frail confidence. The Independent Woman course had made her aware of her tendencies, but, unfortunately, had not offered any hard and fast solutions besides the silly ones, like saying the positive affirmations at her reflection in the mirror She had tried that exercise once, chanting "I am capable. I am confident. I am an Independent Woman," at the mirror, and had felt so stupid that she had stopped almost immediately. So she continued to suffer, perhaps more so knowing the damage she was doing to herself. Now, she forced herself to look at Matt.

He was looking straight ahead, having decided to guide the pair of kayaks himself, to help Kate relax. "How long have you been living in Scottsdale?" he asked.

Okay, an easy one. "A little over three years," Kate answered. "I moved out here from New York."

"*New York, New York,*" Matt crooned. "This must have taken some getting used to." He made a big sweeping gesture with his arm, and Kate assumed he meant the river, the heat, the brown mountains in the distance, the quiet...all of the above.

"It is very different," she agreed. "Have you ever been there?"

"Only once, but after about two days I felt like I had been there forever. It's that kind of place, isn't it?" Kate nodded vigorously. "The one thing I could never figure out," Matt continued, "is when people get any sleep there. I sure as hell didn't get any for about two weeks!"

"Wild days and nights," Kate teased, with a knowing smile. "I've been there." For her, New York was more than home. It was the lifeblood of her soul, a relentless throbbing aura that kept her alive. Or, so she had thought until she moved away. She could now laugh at her old fear of leaving "the city", as she called it; life did exist outside New York. She could somehow see Matt fitting into the New York lifestyle as well as he did out here. Like a chameleon. "Have you always lived here?" she asked him, genuinely interested.

"Arizona, yes; Scottsdale no. I was born near Tucson. Do you know where that is?" Seeing Kate's assent, he added, "I've only just moved to this area, you know. Last week."

Kate felt honored, in a way, that Matt had chosen her, and Jackie, Sam, and George, as his first friends in Scottsdale. "What brought you here? Work?"

Matt nodded. "Of course. I'm a physical education teacher. Junior high kids. You know C. Ramon Junior High School? They've recruited me up from Tucson to do the high school preparation stuff."

Kate was incredulous. "That's where *I* teach!" she exclaimed. "It's really a great place to work. You'll love it. Come to think of it, I did hear a few people talking about a new physical education program to prepare the kids a bit better for high school sports. So you're the one who's going to run that." She shook her head in amazement. "Small world." With the knowledge that Matt would soon be a fellow faculty member at Ramon, he was instantly transported in her mind from the "stranger who happens to be fairly decent" category to that of an ally.

"I haven't been over to the school yet," Matt was saying, "and we start classes in five days. Maybe you could show me around tomorrow, since they'll probably be closed over Labor Day weekend."

Kate nodded. "I'd be happy to show you around Ramon. Luckily, or unluckily, it's not that big. Most of the faculty keep harping on the fact that they didn't take over the adjacent building, as planned. The student population is still growing, although not as rapidly as a couple of years ago, and it does get a bit cramped in some of the classrooms."

"You should have seen the school I just came from, near Tucson. It was built for five hundred students, and when I left in June there were about fifteen hundred. They've got those disgusting looking trailers lined up in front of the main building, and every time they run out of room, they just add another one." He laughed. "I must admit, though, they certainly have made quite a name for themselves in the bilingual education arena. Sometimes I used to think that the Mexican children would walk across the border and just keep walking till they hit Southwest Junior High. Right off the trucks, you know?"

Kate looked puzzled. "I've noticed quite a few Mexicans in my three years here, but I never thought about the implications for schools. You will soon find out there are not that many minorities at Ramon. Maybe about twenty percent."

"In Tucson, I think it is a much more prevalent issue. Being so close to the border. I actually went to night classes to learn Spanish so that I could communicate with some of the immigrant children. I guess I won't have to use it that much here."

Kate sat up in her kayak, impressed. "You can definitely use your Spanish at Ramon. Don't get me wrong. I didn't mean to suggest that there are no Mexican children at the school. There are. But we're an integrated school. We don't cater to those groups. I don't know if I agree with that, but...well, you'll see for yourself when you meet Cooney. That's Alan Coon, the principal."

Matt snickered. "I *have* met him. He was the one who interviewed me last May. And in just over an hour and a half with him, I think I sensed something of what you're talking about. I'm not worried, though. I mean, after all, he did hire me especially to lead up the preparation program. I'm sure he'll let me do my thing." Matt stretched and lay back a little further in his kayak.

The sun had risen to almost its full height in the past hour. It was one of those priceless August days, with just a hint of breeze to sway the leafy trees along the riverbank. A whippoorwill sang its three tones over and over, in a clear ribbon of sound, winding its way downriver, along with the boats.

Kate sighed and looked over at Matt, who was shading his eyes, trying to spot the bird. She wondered for a moment if he was bored with their conversation and contemplated asking him about the wildlife around the river.

"Sometimes it's better to just be still and take in the beauty of nature." Matt's voice shot to the heart of Kate's doubtful mind. She swallowed hard and looked down as he continued,

"A Zen master was walking with a student through the groves of cherry blossom trees. It was springtime, and the student felt it necessary to comment on the beautiful weather and fragrant pink-and-white blossoms. No sooner had he uttered the words when the master gave him a resounding smack on the cheek. The student was shocked. The master, without missing a beat, admonished the student: 'You have disturbed the very beauty that you have been gibbering about. The silence is part of that beauty. Only when your mind can be quiet will you truly appreciate the meaning of what I am saying.'"

Kate felt short of breath and was unable to look at him. She felt exposed and vulnerable, not unlike a child who has been caught doing something bad and scolded. Scoldings had always been so much more painful when her father spoke in that calm tone of voice. At least if he had yelled, she could have gotten angry, yelling back defensively. But as it was, she had felt powerless and ashamed, as if the gentle voice penetrated more deeply into her subconscious to reveal her skinny, naked will. Now, Matt had also found this key to her subconscious. But how, she thought, frustrated...

He read her mind once again, "I can only see other people's thoughts if they want me to. You *did* want me to see them, didn't you?" He paused for her to think and finally shrug her shoulders. "The story about the Zen master, it's pretty powerful, isn't it?" Managing to face him, Kate nodded. "Where did you learn it?" she asked.

"The Zen way of life has been a part of me ever since I spent some time in Japan seven years ago. I don't know how much you know about it, but for me, it has helped to simplify things immensely. I didn't mean anything personal with the story; it's just such a clear way of showing the beauty of silence, don't you think?"

He was trying to draw her out again, smoothing over the rift created by their diverging thoughts. She appreciated his openness and touched his hand briefly. "I'm okay," she smiled. "I would like to know more about the mind-reading, though. Do you have ESP?"

Matt laughed heartily. "I suppose you could call it that, but it's really not anything special. I've read that it is in all of us, and the only reason we can't get to it is that our minds are too cluttered. I've only been able to do it since I began to practice meditation. The quiet mind, you know, that the master was talking about?" He leaned toward her slightly for emphasis and to see if she had understood.

Kate was impressed. "You learned meditation and mind-reading in Japan? I think that's fantastic."

"It's not exactly mind-reading, Kate. It's just being especially tuned into someone else. For example, I could sense you really wanted to know how I was feeling about the silence between us. I *did* kind of want to freak you out, though, and for that I apologize. Sometimes I am a bit of a show-off." He lowered his head and pouted sheepishly.

It seemed inconceivable that this superbly confident person had a streak of humility which somehow blended perfectly into his charming personality. With his head down like that, he reminded her a little of Mitch, her exhusband. There were times when she had felt so exasperated with him that she wanted to throw something at him. Mitch had a way of getting under her skin and bothering her like no one else on earth. She found it extraordinary that the person she loved enough to marry, with his natural exuberance, could turn into such an ogre after a few too many drinks.

Love, hate, love, hate. Her feelings for Mitch used to swing like a pendulum, always one step behind his last change of temperament. And then, just when the frustration level was driving Kate to the limit of her patience, he would look at her with those sad eyes and apologize. Why, why did she always give in and take him into her arms like a lost child? The scene was always the same: the fear, the tears, the vows and caresses and then, sometimes, the lovemaking. It used to give her a temporary sense of security. After all, he still had those qualities that she had fallen in love with. But the pain...it was too much after a while.

Kate squinted to remember the way one day something in her mind snapped and she knew that she could never again take Mitch into her arms and smooth it all over, make it all right again. Strange, how once she had decided, the fear lifted and the hope started seeping back in. Then she couldn't bear to look at Mitch's face when he came to her, full of remorse and promises. In her mind, she was gone already.

Something switched Kate back into the present. It was Matt, splashing droplets of water on her. "I wish I could get rid of that arrogance," he said, shaking his head slowly, more pensive than angry.

She reached over and tousled his hair. "Don't worry. I accept the apology, and I definitely liked the story. It's true that people in general talk too much." As if to prove her point, she closed her eyes and sat back in the kayak again, this time unconcerned about the silence. They drifted down the river to the sound of the whippoorwills and other birds who made the river their home.

After some time, it was Matt who spoke first. "I do love this feeling, though. Don't you?" The sun caught his eyes just then and they shone like brilliant topaz.

Kate nodded. She wasn't sure what she would say if she decided to open her mouth and speak again.

"It's the gliding through the water that does it for me. It's almost like we're one with the boat. You can imagine how a fish feels as it makes its way downriver." She didn't appear ready to comment. He regarded her with an open smile and changed the subject. "You're obviously quite athletic, aren't you?"

She looked at him in amusement. "I try to stay in shape. Kayaking is not really my sport, though I am enjoying it." Small giggle.

"What is your sport?"

"Long-distance running. Although I don't do it competitively anymore." She didn't know why she felt obliged to explain. "I find it so enjoyable to run really hard down a long stretch of flat desert without another soul around."

"I know what you mean. The desert is my favorite place on earth. Most people don't understand what I mean - all they see is a hot, dry, dusty place. But they haven't opened their eyes and seen the beauty of the cactus in flower, or the way the mountains form such a startling dark backdrop with all those mysterious craggy ridges."

"Especially at sunset," Kate added, excitedly.

"Especially anytime," he countered with a conspiratorial smile.

A pins-and-needles sensation rose up the back of Kate's neck and down her arms. She had never before felt such a feeling of kinship with someone. Soul-mates, that's what it felt like. She almost believed she had known Matt in a previous life or something. The whippoorwill called out to them again in its exquisite clear tones. Kate sighed happily, trying to remember why she had resented Matt so much the day before. But yesterday was already so distant, and nothing mattered at all except this perfect moment.

When the rapids got stronger, they took out their paddles

and stroked on either side of the double kayak. A narrow portion of the river was approaching and Matt deftly untied the knot that had kept the boats together for the majority of the outing. With a quick wave, he pushed off from Kate's kayak and sped ahead over the swift current. Kate followed close behind, breathing in the cool spray of the water droplets all around her. When they reached Paw Junction, fifteen minutes later, they found the others, also recently arrived, dragging their kayaks onto the shore, where the rental agency would pick them up and take them back to their car.

Jackie ran over to hug Kate. "Wasn't that sublime?" she breathed. "How is it that we never did this last summer or the summer before?" Without waiting for an answer, she ran to find George, who was opening some bottles of beer.

Kate took an extra minute to touch Matt on the shoulder and say, "Thanks." He wrinkled his nose at her, slightly embarrassed, and they joined the others cooling off in the shade.

Her mood was considerably better than before they had set out, Kate noticed happily. Instead of stifling her, the sun was now caressing her with a gentle heat. But they were only out of the water twenty minutes when George suggested they go back in to cool off.

"I don't know. What about the van?" Ever practical, Jackie glanced at her watch worriedly.

"We have a few minutes," George chided her. "Besides, it will be good to cool off before we have to ride in a hot van for a half hour." And without a moment's hesitation, he picked Jackie up and dropped her into the water.

She splashed armfuls of water at him in mock annoyance, but he had already plunged underwater.

Following suit, Sam made a lunge for Kate.

"No, you don't!" she screamed. "I'll go in on my own, thank you."

Where the sun hit Matt's blond hair, it shone brightly. He looked dubious about entering the river. "You go ahead," he urged Sam, who was waiting for him expectantly.

But as Sam started towards the river, he suddenly turned and picked Matt up in a fireman's lift. Matt appeared to struggle, but Sam maintained his hold on him and soon the two were immersed in the cool water.

Treading water, she watched this scene in amusement. "You didn't put up too much of a fight," she teased Matt in a quiet voice, when he bobbed to the surface right next to her.

He shrugged. "I didn't mind either way, but he seemed to want me in here, so here I am."

Matt began to tread water about three feet away from her and the small ripples he made kept moving towards her and disappearing into her own circle of ripples. Mesmerized by the smooth motion, Kate felt content and at peace. She knew that Matt's eyes were on her and she wanted to return his look, but the water held her in a trance-like state, suspended in time.

Just as he was about to make a move towards Kate, he heard the shouting behind him.

"You can't keep up with me," George called out as he swam faster in the direction of the shore. He left Jackie far behind, although she splashed choppily forward in an effort to reach George.

"Wait, George." Her voice came in a pant. "I have a pain in my side."

"No sympathy, babe," George yelled. "I didn't tell you to drink all that beer." He was almost at the water's edge.

Jackie struck out at the water like a propeller sputtering to get started. She sucked in a mouthful of water and coughed harshly. "Come on, George." Her voice was now more of a whimper as she pleaded for him to wait.

It didn't occur to Matt to stay where he was. With smooth strokes, his arms cut through the water until he reached Jackie's flailing form. "I think he won," he joked, as he swam up to her. "Just grab onto my shoulder if you feel tired." He left it as an option, not wanting to embarrass her by assuming that she needed help.

Gratefully, Jackie placed her hand on Matt's shoulder and he guided her closer to the shore, where her feet could touch the bottom.

Having observed all this like someone watching a silent film in slow motion, Sam finally came to life and joined Matt and Jackie. "Hey, are you all right?"

"Of course she is," Matt answered for her. "I just showed her who's boss, that's all."

On the surface, his tone was full of mischief, but he kept his eye on Jackie, saw that her breathing had slowed to a normal rate. "And none too soon, I can see. The van's just pulled up to take us back to the cars."

There wasn't time to say anything else as they all clambered up onto the dirt to get ready for the trip back. Jackie sidled up to George, who, having realized what had almost happened, was overcome with worry after the fact. He had his arm around her protectively and he carried all of their gear.

"Well," Kate stated to no one in particular. "I guess it's time to go." She moved slowly, transfixed by the shock. Out of the corner of her eye, she saw Matt hoist one of the kayaks onto his shoulder and her heart skipped a beat. He looked so beautiful, even with his matted-down river-water hair. She felt a strong pull towards him, which she carefully placed to one side as she climbed into the van with the others. *Don't fall too hard for this guy*, something inside her warned. *You can't handle it.*

Chapter 3

C. Ramon Junior High School exemplified the best Spanish architecture of its time, having been built almost a hundred years earlier, when missionaries still had as their mission to convert all heathens to Christianity. Originally a general school for all children between the ages of four and fourteen, the numbers eventually grew too large for the sprawling one-story stucco building, and it was decided that the younger students would go to an elementary school down the road.

The 1950's and 60's had brought further growth to the old school. With an influx of baby-boomers, an expansion project had been taken on by the local board of education, funded by a donation from a prosperous graduate of the school, Carlos Ramon. Desiring to see his name live on in the Phoenix area where so many of his relatives made their home, Ramon made his gift conditional on the fact that the renovated building be named after him. And so it was that C. Ramon Junior High School bore the name of a Mexican whose grandfather had been one of the first to benefit from the mission's own educational program.

Now, as she and Matt made their way on foot up the long drive, Kate felt proud of the building which had practically been her home for the past three years. The second story added a certain elegance, she thought, as well as the red ceramic tiles on the roof. Although the teachers' parking lot was empty on this last Friday morning before the new school year, Kate had parked as far away from the building as possible, to give Matt the full impact of the whitewashed stucco, gleaming in the sun. "After all," she said, "you will only see it for the first time once." Matt nodded enthusiastically as they approached the school.

They entered via the side door, to which all full-time teachers had a key. The effect of the cool dark hallway was a powerful one for Kate, who had managed to stay away all summer. She stopped for a moment to breathe in the smell of the tile floor, mingled with chalk dust and wooden desks. It was a familiar smell, not really different from that of her old school in New York. It had, well, that education smell, which acted like a salve to her frenetic emotional state. Yes, this was where she belonged.

Matt, sensing Kate's need to make contact again with the building, had moved down the hallway somewhat, feeling the coolness of the walls, and trying to take in the rest of the aura. Kate came up behind him slowly and led the way. "I'm glad there's no one here today." Her voice echoed slightly in the empty corridor. "Although I love it when it's buzzing with kids and teachers."

"Teaching in a place like this has been my dream for many years, ever since I decided to become a teacher. I actually went to an elementary school very similar to this one near Tucson. I imagined there were ghosts still roaming the halls, left over from the Wild West days."

"How long have you wanted to be a teacher?" Kate asked, feeling more than ever a sense of kinship with him.

"Ever since the fifth grade, when I had a superb teacher named Brother Michael. It was a monastery school, you see. Brother Michael must have been one of the monks that founded the school, he was so old. But the kindest teacher you ever met. He was one of the few Catholics I've met that actually practiced what he preached. Patience, honesty, charity, Brother Michael showed us the meaning of these things with his actions, rather than sermons."

This statement was delivered in a sharp tone, which made Kate wonder about the underlying meaning of Matt's words. But there was no time to mention it because they had arrived at the big metal door which led to the gymnasium, Matt's new domain. She pulled the door open, allowing him to enter the cavernous room first. This was one of the improvements that had been made with Ramon's gift, and there seemed to have been nothing omitted. Ropes, beams, and bars all stood in perfect array, while two trampolines leaned against the far wall. Cages with locked covers displayed bats, balls of all sizes, and various nets, folded neatly and stacked, ready for any sport.

Nodding once, Matt said, "Yep. This is what he promised. Everything ready to go; now it's just up to me." He took it all in one more time, then motioned for them to leave. "Come on, I want to see where you do your thing."

Kate's classroom was housed on the second floor, with the other English teachers and foreign language teachers. She had been able to keep the same room as last year, which had saved her the headache of moving everything out, as she had done the previous year. She had viewed this as a small win, a sign of approval from Cooney, who was the bane of their existence at Ramon. Opening the door with her key, she noticed that apart from the clean floor and furniture, everything was pretty much the same as when she had left it in June. There were even two shrivelled balloons on the corner of her desk to remind her of the end-of-year festivities she had enjoyed with the students.

"This is it," Kate said with a small laugh, hoping the room spoke for itself. "Just looks like an empty hull now, but it's usually packed. I haven't heard the final numbers yet, but Cooney usually gives me more students than I handle effectively, and then it's a struggle for space. Not to mention individual attention. But he can't seem to say no to the PTA. 'Oh, really, Kate,'" she mimicked, "'what's one more student?' That's his attitude, but he doesn't see that's it's always 'just one more'. But never mind all that. It shouldn't affect you." Jutting her chin out slightly, she left the classroom with Matt.

That evening, Kate was blowing on a tray of cookies, trying to cool them, so she could lift them onto a plate. She wanted to take something homemade to Matt's house, since he had invited her over for a home-cooked dinner. She rushed out the door with the still-warm cookies, and jogged across the walkway. She knocked on the door quite loudly, to be heard over the music that was pouring out of every window.

"Come around to the living room," Matt's voice made itself heard over the music, which was then lowered to a decent level. "Sorry," he grinned sheepishly. "The spicier the dish, the louder the music I play while I'm cooking, to get myself psyched up." Seeing her eyes widen, he laughed uncontrollably. Wiping his eyes with the corner of an apron, he finally spluttered, "I'm only kidding. Of course, growing up so close to the Mexican border, I know how to make a mean chili, but I wouldn't do that to you. Not unless you want me to."

Relaxing into a low leather chair, Kate waved him away with a hand. "Whatever you're serving, I'm sure it's delicious." And it was. It was one of the best Mexican meals she had ever had, on either coast. As they were clearing the dishes from the table, she asked him where he had learned to cook like that.

"Oh, here and there," he answered, "but mostly from watching my mother. She is a big believer in equal rights, especially since that means I could give her a hand when I lived at home. Trying to take care of five kids and a household is quite a handful."

"Five kids!" Kate exclaimed. "I don't know any families with that many children. It must have been so much fun growing up."

"Well, actually," explained Matt, "it was very well organized. My mother dished out a fair bit of responsibility along with her cooking. And as the oldest, I got the most. But I wouldn't have it any other way," he concluded, protectively.

Kate was shaking her head in amazement. Her ideas about this newcomer kept changing with each new aspect of him that was revealed. Although she still found him flippant, she was beginning to discover a deeper side to him, a core of meaning and experience that ran through him, like a jagged vein of iron lode unearthed during a blast. His experiences seemed too fantastic to be real: Japan, a monastery school, four younger brothers and sisters...suddenly it occurred to Kate that Matt could be a pathological liar. She listened more closely as he continued.

"You don't get a lot of privacy," he said slowly. "I'm pretty good at sharing, but when I wanted my time alone, I had to escape on long walks in the desert." He sighed.

"I always wished I had a brother or sister...."

"Yeah, all in all, the five of us are really close and I would do anything for my brothers and sisters. Absolutely anything." This was said in an ultra-serious tone.

"Anyway, one of my sisters will actually be coming up here

in a few weeks, to look at colleges. I'll introduce you to her then."

Reassured that he was telling the truth, Kate asked him if he managed to stay close to his family, despite the distance and disparate lifestyles.

"We're extremely close, my family." He sounded almost defensive. "It's all you have in the end, really. I think people in the West take their families for granted; they certainly don't value their parents or brothers and sisters the way they do in the East." He shook his head in disbelief.

"But your parents aren't from the Far East, are they?" She was puzzled. He didn't have an Oriental look about him, but there could be some other explanation, maybe.

He shook his head slowly. "Not exactly. Although my father spent a lot of time over there with his job. I think it had a big effect on him, in fact I know it did. He became very friendly with a Japanese family while he was on an assignment over there and they treated him like their own son. Wonderful people, the Kato family."

"And your mother?" Kate was genuinely interested and she hoped it didn't sound too much like Twenty Questions.

"Oh, my mother is just a saint. She went to Japan with my father many times before we were born and then a couple of times we all went. My mother understood the deeper level on which my father harbored his feelings for Japan. She never lost her patience with him, even though she had to listen to hours upon hours of his stories. She even encouraged him to write about it. I'm lucky, I was able to spend a few months in Japan one summer. It was then that I really started to see what the attraction for my father had always been."

Matt gazed off in the distance and Kate wondered whether he would continue. Finally, he spoke in a softer voice. "My mother has always taught us the importance of being close, being there for each other." There was a slight pause as Matt cleared his throat. "It's been especially important since my father died."

"Oh. I didn't know. I'm sorry to hear that." So inadequate, so wooden the words sounded, but she felt it necessary to say something.

He motioned to her empty coffee cup, but she shook her head. "No, thanks. You are lucky, Matt, to have had such a diverse background and to have been exposed to so much while you were growing up." The images were still whirling around in her head as she pictured the Kato family showing Matt's father, and then Matt, the culture of their country. How she would love to visit Japan...

"How about you, Kate? What was it like growing up with all of your parents' attention? You're not spoiled, are you?" he teased.

"No!" she answered indignantly. "It's taught me a lot about fending for myself, that's for sure." She felt funny, as though she was trying to justify her situation. The more she thought about her relationship with her parents, the worse she began to feel. Because she was, indeed, a prime example of what Matt had been condemning just minutes earlier: she took her parents for granted, they hardly called each other, hardly saw each other. Hell, she hardly even thought about them, so wrapped up was she in her new life in Arizona. Yes, they had taught her to be independent, but she yearned for the close-knit family unit Matt was describing. There was no way she wanted to get into this with her new friend.

He seemed to understand because he didn't press any further. He gathered Yellowstone's big, furry body onto his lap and smoothed the top of the dog's head as he spoke. "I hope you don't think I am some fanatic who's infatuated with Japan and hates America. Because I don't. There are great things about both cultures. I'll probably always have both of them inside me. I don't know if you follow me."

"I do," she nodded. "At least, I think I do."

Matt chortled. "Don't worry. Maybe some day I can take you to Japan and show you why it is so special."

The idea of it made her catch her breath. She didn't dare say a word. She knew in that instant that she would go anywhere with Matt, would do anything for him. She didn't know why she felt so certain of this, but as she let out a long, relaxed breath, she knew it more strongly than she had ever known anything else in her life.

"Hey," Matt murmured. "It's late, buddy." He got up and stretched with a loud grunt. Somehow, it was two-twenty in the morning, so they bade each other good night, promising to see each other sometime over the long weekend. Kate was home one minute later.

The next morning, the sun pried Kate out of bed with its rays reaching all the way into her bedroom onto the waterbed. She stretched, knowing that if she rolled over, she would just fall back asleep again. She rubbed her eyes and remembered the Desert Botanical Gardens. *Okay*, she commanded her body, *up! Now!*

She dressed hurriedly, noticing the time was later than she had hoped to wake up. The Botanical Gardens was one place where Kate could go and see all around her the Arizona flora that she loved. The Gardens contained more species of cactus than even she could recognize, although she did her best to learn as much as possible about the strange, prickly plants.

Inexplicable, possibly, but ever since Kate had moved out here to Arizona, she had been fascinated by the desert plants that survived on so little water and thrived in temperatures that practically boiled human blood. *Well, maybe not so inexplicable*, she mused, thinking for the hundredth time how similar a cactus plant was to a human being. So tough on the outside, sharp, hurting those around him, but strong, strong, strong. A real survivor. When cut, the plant revealed a soft inside, with enough juice to live on. It could feed off itself for months, until the next rainfall. Just like a person finding the strength inside to make it through the hard times...

Kate stopped herself before she let her mind dwell on the "hard times". Yes, she had suffered, but here she was, in sunny Arizona, learning to live again. She bolted out the door in an effort to shed the mood and plunge into the beautiful day. On an impulse, she wandered over to Matt's house. Normally, she liked to be alone in the Botanical Gardens, using the time to think, but Matt had been so nice to cook dinner that she felt like reciprocating. Besides, he had probably never seen the displays of natural wonder at the Gardens.

As she approached Matt's place and was just about to ring the bell, she saw a figure out of the corner of her eye. Matt was around the side of the house, on the grass, and he appeared to be doing a slow-motion type of karate. Kate stopped dead in her tracks, not wanting to disturb him, although she was at least fifty feet away. She stood there, motionless, watching him go through the exotic movements of arms, hands, and legs. When he turned around suddenly and came toward her, she instantly wished she had not stood gaping like that, intruding on his privacy. But it was too late to turn around or pretend she had not seen him.

"Good morning!" Matt yelled, unconcerned about waking the neighbors. "Did you sleep well?"

"I slept like a baby. There must have been something in that salsa." She worried that she had interrupted his routine. "You can get back to whatever that was you were doing. I was just going to see if you wanted to join me on an outing to the Desert Botanical Gardens. But don't let me keep you." Kate felt the familiar sensation of words pouring out of her mouth in a rapid, endless stream and clamped her lips together quickly.

"Oh, my kata." Matt smiled easily. "I've just finished my morning routine. Did you like it?"

"Yes," breathed Kate, "but what exactly is it you were doing? 'Kata', did you say?" She was certain it was something Oriental, but rather than pretend like she usually did, she was genuinely curious to know more about it.

"Yes. They're karate exercises, the basic movements broken down into distinct parts. Individual movements are strung together purposefully yet, hopefully, smoothly, to form the entire kata. But actually, the real meaning of kata is more like 'how one behaves'.[1] Precision is everything, you see." To illustrate, he executed a sharp cut through the air with his right hand, while jumping up and landing deftly on both feet. "Can you picture it?" His eyes sparkled.

Then he saw that Kate was standing perfectly still with her mouth slightly agape. "Oh, God, I'm sorry for babbling." He shook his head. "I'm sorry," he said again. "I don't remember sometimes that not everyone gets as excited about it as I do."

"Don't be silly," she argued. "I'm fascinated. Where did you learn that?"

"When I started taking karate fifteen years ago, you know, one of those tykes running around in the white cotton robe and pants?"

How could he make light of everything? Kate shook her head. "Fifteen years," she said aloud. "Surely you must be a black belt or something."

Here Matt let out a loud guffaw. "I didn't say that I kept it up for fifteen years. Not seriously anyway. Mostly I did it for the discipline, and the kata are good exercises to keep that going, even if I never do anything else." He cast his eyes downward and mumbled, "I did get my brown belt, though. But that was eight years ago. God knows if I could ever compete seriously now." His serious frown made a deep furrow in the middle of his brow.

Kate could feel his unwillingness to say any more about the karate and wondered if she should mention the Botanical Gardens again.

"I could be ready in about ten minutes if the offer still stands?" Matt pre-empted her question.

He ran inside to get changed while she waited on the front step, trying to tan her face. It puzzled her, his nonchalance mixed with that reticence, but she knew better than to pry. From what she could see, Matt was just exceptionally talented, multi-talented. She wished she had more of the natural ability that seemed to emanate from him. *Let it go*, she reminded herself sternly, and returned her attention to the mid-morning rays.

As they walked slowly through the Gardens, each was caught up in his private experience of the plants, yet still aware of the other's presence. Matt lingered at the flowering cacti, marvelling at their ability to blossom in such harsh surroundings. He let himself become absorbed by their simplicity, enraptured even.

Ecstatic that Matt was enjoying the plants as much as she was, Kate felt all tension slip off her body like a silken robe. She was glad there was no need to talk, since she never could have explained the feelings that arose when in the presence of these plants. The Gardens never let her down; they proclaimed their peace to her, allowing her to enter into it effortlessly. How different this was from the "real world" of the school, her neighbors, and even friends. Here, there was no presumption, no expectation, and Kate drank it in, knowing that in just two days the spell would be broken, and routine would take over.

Chapter 4

Crumpled papers and empty cans were scattered all over the floor of the classroom, and Kate felt defeated, as though she had failed again in her duty. She knew the cleaning people could just as easily take care of the litter, but her sense of pride would not allow her to leave it there; it would most certainly be a reflection on her, on her inability to control her class. Despite repeated reminders about picking up after themselves, the students of American Literature 201 were not responding.

Maybe, Kate pondered, as she sat down wearily at a desk, *maybe they don't want to be mothered and maybe I shouldn't try.* But, why did they have to be so sloppy? Didn't they have any manners? She didn't know why it even bothered her so much.

A loud bang made her start. Matt had entered her classroom and dropped his bag on her desk. "Ready?" he grinned, his eyes wild like a tiger ready to pounce.

Giggling, Kate pointed a finger at him. "If you scare me to death, I won't be in any shape to go anywhere." She had planned a spontaneous outing to a local bar for happy hour, inviting seven or eight other teachers, including Matt. Normally, she would have waited for someone else to plan something, but she was feeling particularly alive and capable, and she wanted to introduce Matt to the others, so that he could make friends.

Over the past three days since classes had started, she had hardly seen Matt, since he was usually in the gym and she in her classroom upstairs.

Once, they had bumped into each other in the staff lounge, where Matt had been arm wrestling with another male teacher, with a small crowd of onlookers cheering them on. Kate felt certain that he would get along fabulously with the other teachers, but she still wanted to help him get to know the others in an informal setting.

"Okay," she said, jumping up and throwing the last few cans in the garbage can by the door. "It's off to Shorty's." Shorty's was the local sports bar-cum-"pickup joint". The Ramon staff tended to hang out there after school because it was close and the drinks were cheap. Shorty, the amiable, moustached proprietor, had designated the hours between three o'clock and five o'clock "Ramon Happy Hour" and the teachers were grateful.

Inside the bar, three or four teachers were already gathered around a tall, round table, drinks in hand. With the exception of two flannel-clad regulars with four bottles of Budweiser lined up on their table in the back, the Ramon representatives were the only customers in the bar.

"So let me get this straight," Eddie Price was saying, leaning over the table and pushing his face into Harry Carp's. "They can pour over the border in droves, practically trampling on each other to get here, moving into our neighborhoods and making property values plummet, with their millions of dirty children and dogs, and then we're expected to make them feel at home by offering them an entire program in Spanish!" He spat these last two words at Carp and shook his head emphatically.

Oh, no, Kate groaned inwardly. *Not again.* The age-old question of bilingual education usually reared its ugly head at least once in every gathering, but generally not this early in the conversation. Kate suspected, from the aroma of stale beer coming from the table, as well as Eddie's slight stagger, that the small group of teachers had been able to leave Ramon at two-thirty and had been drinking for the past hour, at least. Kate started as a cold bottle brushed her arm.

Matt thrust the Mexican beer into her hand and started over to the table of teachers.

"Just to warn you," Kate whispered, grabbing on to his sleeve, "they are going at it again on the bilingual issue. If you want to sit over there instead, that's fine with me." She hoped Matt would choose the adjacent table, where they could sit and enjoy their beers until some of their other, less fanatical, colleagues arrived.

Matt was continuing toward Eddie's table. He gave a general wave at the group and they immediately made room for him and Kate to sit down. After the general introductions (Matt had met most of the teachers within the past few days anyway), Eddie leaned over the table again, poised to continue his argument where he had left off.

"These bozos," he snarled, by way of an explanation, "think that we should spend the taxpayers' hard-earned money on developing a Spanish program to cater to the Mexican immigrant children."

"Now, hang on, Eddie," interrupted Mary Sinclair. "Some of us actually agree with you, if you would just shut up for a minute and let us talk. You see," she addressed Matt, "the program would cost about three million dollars to develop, not to mention the staff changes and building renovations. We'd certainly have to expand to accommodate the influx of kids that would be involved in such a program." She smiled benignly. "For the Board of Education to make any decisions at all is like getting a rock to piss." The entire table exploded into hysterical laughter at Mary's mixed-up analogy.

Matt used the break as his entrée. "Actually, the school where I used to teach has one of the best bilingual education programs in the nation. I happen to think that it's an excellent idea, when administered properly." Nobody said anything, so he continued, "I've seen many Mexican children start school without knowing any English at all and within two months be nearly caught up with their classmates, enough at least for them to be placed in a normal class."

"Yeah, so, we have Mexicans and several other minorities at Ramon, and the kids do just fine." Eddie had recovered his voice and was prepared to turn the discussion into a fight again.

Matt remained nonplussed. "I have no doubt that those children who actually make it past the administration manage all right, but what about the ones who never get in because their English isn't good enough?" His mild tone conveyed no hard feelings, but, as he looked around the table, he truly expected an answer from someone. There was none.

Mary Sinclair finally spoke up again. "Matt, the ideals may be great, and I have no doubt that if we had the money we might be in a different frame of mind. But we don't. And, personally, I would like to see us use the adjacent building for an art studio and proper auditorium. It would cost a lot less money, that's for sure." Feeling pleased with herself, Mary took a sip of her beer. Having worked at Ramon for eleven years, she was one of the senior members of staff, and her opinions were generally taken seriously by the others.

"How many of us speak Spanish?" The answer to the question, seemingly innocent enough, would give Matt more ammunition, Kate knew.

She could feel his argument gaining momentum like a silent volcano bubbling underneath the earth.

Only Matt and Harry Carp had their hands up. Harry moved his arm to half-mast, while mumbling, "Well, I can get by. I wouldn't say I'm fluent."

"That's fine, that's fine," encouraged Matt, patting him on the back. "Enough to get by, that's all I'm talking about. You see, if we can't even communicate with them, how are we supposed to know what it is they want or need?"

"Who *cares* what they want or need!" Eddie's face was red and his eyes bulging. "They moved to *this* country, godammit, and they take what they get!" He glared around the table, while everyone else sat frozen in horror.

Kate felt sorry for Matt, whose first impression of her coworkers and friends was turning out so negative. But he was just sitting in his chair, with a contemplative look on his face, trying to understand Eddie Price's point of view. He nodded his head knowingly.

"Oh, well, it probably won't change the way they run around the bases," he remarked with a light laugh, although even as he said it, he recalled some coaching he had done in Spanish, to help some of the more recent arrivals at his old school to improve their batting stances.

"You're right, buddy," Harry Carp jumped in here, thankful for the chance to end the controversial discussion. Head of the debate team, Harry admired Matt's grace in steering the conversation toward a more acceptable topic. He made a mental note to talk to Matt at a later date about helping out with the team.

An hour later, the group was clinking glasses to Ramon's future, their own sanity, and even the formidable principal, Alan Coon. Kate was debating whether or not to have a third beer when she saw Sam enter the bar. "Sam!" she yelled, realizing that it had been a while since she had seen him.

Sam strode over to the table of teachers, most of whom he knew at least by sight. He greeted them cordially, but declined the chair that was being proffered. "I'm meeting George here in a few minutes, thanks. Nice to see you though." As he turned to find another, smaller table, he bent down to whisper in Kate's ear, "You're looking beautiful, as usual. Stop by and say hi sometime, okay?"

As Kate watched his retreating back, she felt enormously guilty for having neglected her friends over the past week. She had not seen them except in passing since the day of the kayaking; all her spare time had been spent with Matt. With a mumbled apology to the table, Kate went over to join Sam.

"How have you been, anyway?" She really wanted to know, and hoped that Sam would not become sarcastic out of jealousy.

Sam replied that he was fine, work was fine, and that he missed seeing her. There was a depth to his voice that Kate had never heard before, and his dark eyes were searching, longing to say more, although he remained silent.

Kate did not want to get into a serious talk with Sam now, in the bar, with everyone at the next table. She bit her lip and smiled back at Sam, doubts festering in her overactive mind. Luckily, George was just coming into the room, and Kate felt relieved not to have to answer Sam's unspoken question.

Ever the clown, George pretended to sit down on Kate's

knee, while putting only about half his weight down. "I want to ride the horsey, Mommy," he pleaded.

"Get off," Kate laughed. "It's good to see you, George. What's new?" As she listened to George talk about the promotion he was trying to get at his company, she was aware that her concentration was not as it should be; rather, she kept looking over to the table where Matt was still sitting with the other teachers, playing some silly drinking game. Sam's hand landed on her own which was wrapped around a glass. She glanced quickly at him, startled. "Kate's a little distracted," he explained to George. The tone was mild, but Kate was concerned that there was something else behind the words. She couldn't read anything at all behind Sam's dark eyes.

This isn't fair, she frowned to herself. She and Sam had always had a very open relationship. He had been one of her first friends in Arizona, filling a very big gap until Jackie had moved out to join her. His contemplative nature had helped her work through the remainder of her trauma and put it behind her.

Sam had complimented her last year about helping him open up. Had said she was the only one who had gotten through his super-tough shell, to the sensitive man underneath. She didn't recall doing anything special; in fact, she had felt honored that he had shared as much with her as he had. He had taken her to the Navajo reservation where he had been born, and where his family still lived. She laughed to herself as she remembered his sister telling her she was the first girl Sam had brought home to meet his parents, and how worried she had been that this marked something 'official', something she was not ready for.

Nonsense, Sam had assured her on their return to Scottsdale. His parents didn't control what he did anyway. And they had been friendly towards her, organizing an impromptu tour of the reservation for her.

Yes, ever since then, Sam had seemed even closer to her, since he had obviously shared an important part of himself with her. He began to tell Kate the story of his breaking away from his roots and exploring a new way of life, opening up to her as she had to him only months earlier. Had that door closed shut since then? And could it be pried open again?

"I'm not distracted," she defended herself now, with a slight pout. She made an extra effort to pay attention. "Good luck with the interview, George. You deserve it, if anyone does. Always working those long hours."

George shifted his weight in his chair. "Thanks for the vote of confidence, but I don't think it looks too good, babe. There are a couple of others that have been on the project a lot longer than I have. But there are a couple of other opportunities I'm looking at just in case."

She raised an eyebrow at him. "What? What?" she prompted when he said nothing.

"Oh no." George shared a conspiratorial smile with Sam. "Top secret. Sorry, but you'll be one of the first to know if it works out." In typical George style, he brushed off the important matter and changed the subject. "Is Mr. Popularity going to come over here and join us for a drink?" He indicated toward Matt.

Seeing them looking in his direction, he motioned that he would be over shortly. He joined them after a short discourse with the bartender on the joys of a perfect margarita. As the men chatted happily about their respective jobs and frustrations, Kate stayed relatively quiet, observing how easily Matt had fit in to the two groups that were so much a part of her life. Meanwhile, with Eddie and Harry gone home and Mary nursing one of Matt's "perfect margaritas", the large group dispersed and Kate invited Mary to join her friends from Sunny Vista.

"I never get picked up in this place," Mary said, after the introductions had been performed. "Maybe we should find another hang-out."

"You want to get picked up, Mary?" Matt asked. Before she could answer, Matt had jumped up and lifted Mary off her seat effortlessly. He put her back down carefully on the chair and wiped his hands on his pants. "There. Now, you can't tell me you've never gotten picked up at Shorty's."

All three men hooted in glee, Kate was shocked. But Mary, a wry smile on her face, leaned close to Matt's face and said, "That was the quickest quickie I've ever had, too. I didn't even break a sweat." More laughter. Touché, Mary.

With her sardonic wit, Mary proceeded to tell them stories of the old days at Ramon. She added a spark to the conversation that seemed to ignite the others, and Kate felt satisfied that she had pulled together a successful event. She allowed herself to be carried away on the tide of peace that seemed to permeate the entire bar, the Friday afternoon slowing-down of a clock that had been ticking much too fast during the week.

Chapter 5

The wiry teenager jumped down from the parallel bars for the third time in five minutes. He sighed heavily, wiped his palms in the box of chalk dust, and returned to face Matt. "I don't know what it is, Mister Reynolds," the boy said, then shrugged his shoulders, at a loss for words. He was concentrating very hard, and saw a gradual improvement, but certainly not enough to qualify for Ramon's gymnastics team.

Matt put his hands on Pedro Morales' shoulders. He spoke slowly, making sure not to reprimand the boy. "That was actually very good, Pedro. We just need to get you a bit straighter before the lift. Maybe it would help if you could look straight ahead instead of at the bar. You know where the bar is; you don't need to look at it. Just look straight." He gazed upwards, searching for the word. "*Derecho!*" he exclaimed, looking to Pedro for confirmation. "*Mira derecho y no a la barra.*"

Pedro smiled broadly, appreciative. He nodded his head enthusiastically and went over to the bars again.

Kate, from her perch on the bleachers, applauded silently. She definitely approved of this way of teaching that Matt had, especially the patient individual approach designed to help each athlete reach his personal objective. Kate knew that

Matt's approach took extra time, and that he often stayed on, working with students until six or seven in the evening. As long as the kids were willing to work with him, he would be there for them. Some of the students Matt coached were varsity athletes, desperate to improve their performance against other schools' players. Others had personal goals to achieve, such as climbing the ropes all the way to the ceiling or making their way around the 800-yard track. Requiring additional coaching were those students who had been classified by the athletics authority as "uncoordinated". It was a term that had stuck with them ever since the qualification tests, and would continue to stick with them for the duration of their public education. Worst of all, these students were not included in the general physical education classes with the other students; instead, they were given special exercises to work on during the gym period, exercises that would supposedly improve their coordination.

"They never get proper coaching," Matt had complained to Kate several weeks ago as they had hiked up one of the mountains near the development in the late afternoon. "And without proper coaching, they will never 'catch up' with the other students." He had proceeded to explain to Kate the bureaucracy of physical education programs in public schools, stopping with every major point to gesture emotionally. Kate had listened attentively, not having realized until that day what a political minefield the issue was. Matt's commitment, as he explained it that day against the backdrop of the setting sun, was to help each student, no matter what his or her present level or capability, to improve and reach the next level.

As Matt directed his attention to Pedro Morales' technique on the parallel bars, the sunset conversation echoed in Kate's ears, complementing the dedication she was witnessing. She felt momentarily transported to a higher plane, and the feeling made her slightly lightheaded with excitement. Most of the teachers at Ramon were good at what they did, but this level of personal attachment to one's work was seldom seen. Kate made a mental promise to be more patient with her students, and to help those that were having trouble keeping up.

In Kate's car on the way home, there was a calm glowing feeling, as though both she and Matt had run a few miles around the track. Basking in this calm, Kate realized she wanted to be around Matt that evening, to prevent it from dissipating. *I'm addicted*, she thought to herself, more amused than surprised. She offered to cook dinner, and Matt quickly agreed, not in the mood to do much cooking for himself. During the past three weeks, they had enjoyed three or four dinners at Kate's house; Matt said he was keeping score so that he could reciprocate some day. The truth was that it was easier to go to Kate's and she seemed able to whip up a meal more quickly than he could. "The gourmet banquet, that's my forte," he was fond of saying.

Satiated after the spaghetti dinner, Kate reclined back into the softness of the leather sofa, balancing her wineglass on her knee. She looked through the pink tint at Matt and laughed at the distorted image.

"What's so funny?" Matt demanded.

"When I look through this wineglass..." Kate exploded into gales of laughter, unable to finish the sentence.

Matt leaped across the sofa to look through her glass.

"No, no." She pushed him away weakly, still giggling. "How can you look at yourself through my wineglass? You're not even over there now." She gave him an impulsive hug. Suddenly, she realized that he was practically on top of her, and she waded through the wine-induced fog to the present. The sensation was powerful, as though she had been knocked over by a ten-foot wave and was now floating on top of the salty ocean towards the shore. Kate noticed she had been holding her breath and let it out now in a shallow stream. She wanted to kiss him so badly, but felt paralyzed.

Matt leaned across the small gap between them and placed his lips on hers. He cradled her head with one hand and encircled the small of her back with the other. The kiss was long and luxurious, sending shivers up and down Kate's arms and legs. She matched the pressure of his lips, then pulled away gently to kiss the rest of his face. As she reached the broad brow, she could feel Matt's breath on her breasts, and felt a longing for him streaming up through her legs, up to her chest, and finally her neck, leaving her feeling breathless and faint.

Sensing the response in her body, Matt picked her up lightly and lay her down again on the sofa, this time lying next to her. Kate felt the heat of his breath as he caressed her neck with fingertips and lips, each touch becoming more intense. She wanted to scream with relief as his body molded to hers and she felt his hardness through her jeans. Returning the feverish kisses, she became aware of his scent, vaguely familiar and infinitely sexy. Kate pressed herself against his body and stroked his face. Opening her eyes, she saw Matt's own gaze on her, describing his joy and yearning.

A smile, a wave of peace washing over her. Suddenly, she was sobbing uncontrollably, the floodgates having opened with her heart. She lay against Matt, tears soaking his shirt and sobs racking her body. A blurry look at him told her that he was not shocked or horrified, and her gratitude for this sent her into further hysterics. Matt continued to hold her, stroking her back gently and breathing steadily. Slowly, Kate calmed down and began to breathe in time to the rise and fall of Matt's chest. She felt too powerless to speak, although she knew that her was not expecting her to say anything.

Rising from the sofa, Kate whispered that she would be right back, and made her way to the bathroom. The harsh light of the bulbs reflected in the mirror, giving her an objective look at her tear-streaked face. She shook her head at the reflection. *Nice going, Bennett,* she scolded, but she didn't have the heart to continue. She had had enough suffering for one night, she figured, as she splashed cold water on her face and combed her hair. Many similar occasions had taught her the importance of calming down quickly and dousing her eyes with the coldest water she could stand, to bring down the swelling and reduce the redness. Satisfied that her outward appearance no longer conveyed her inner hurt, she emerged from the bathroom.

The doorbell sounded when she was halfway across the living room. She looked at Matt, who had poured himself another glass of wine and was studying one of her poetry books. Taking a deep breath, Kate opened the door.

Sam bounded in. "You'll never believe it!" he shouted dramatically. "Oh, hi, Matt," he added as he noticed him. "You guys are just not going to believe it," he repeated, pausing for effect.

"What, what?" Kate prompted, slightly disoriented by Sam's barging in, but curious to hear what he was so excited about.

"They're moving to Denver. George and Jackie," he explained, noting Kate's blank look. "I knew he was going for the position in Denver, but we were both pretty sure he wouldn't get it. He did, though. Isn't that great? And Jackie, do you believe it, she decided to follow him there. Oh, but surely she must have told you by now." Sam halted this monologue to see if Kate knew any more about it.

She was still recovering from the shock of the news, which had taken her completely by surprise. Jackie had not said anything to her, but then, the two women had hardly seen each other since the school year had begun. Kate felt the guilt like a lump at the bottom of her stomach as she realized how she had neglected her friends. She half-consoled herself by admitting that they had not called her, either.

"When are they going?" Matt asked.

"Next Thursday." Sam's enthusiasm had dribbled away into dejection at the reality of losing a close friend and roommate. Kate herded Sam into the hall, closing the door. "Come on," she said. "We can't stay here in the hall all night. Go sit down over there. White wine all right, or would you prefer coffee?"

"Coffee, please," Sam mumbled. Matt went over to sit with him and Kate prepared the coffee, comfortably moving into the role of hostess. She heard Matt asking Sam about George's decision and hurriedly put the coffee cups and milk onto a tray and returned to the living room.

"Of course, it's great for George. A huge increase in salary and they're paying for everything." He paused to take a sip of coffee. "Thanks, Kate, this is perfect. So, anyway, Jackie decided to go with him. As you know, they're going to get married in the spring anyway." He looked at Kate, expecting her to fill in the details.

"Actually," Kate said, still rather dumbfounded, "Jackie and I haven't seen each other much lately. I've been so busy with classes and everything..." She toyed with the rings on her fingers. This was all happening so fast. She felt a tug of desperation about so few days left with her best friend from back East, and vowed silently to get together with her the following day.

Sam was inviting them to a farewell party he was having the following Wednesday. Kate had to smile. Sam and George had managed to stay in touch with many college friends, most of whom lived within an hour or two of Phoenix and they hosted big get-togethers once or twice a year, inviting all of them. Kate had been to a few of these parties and she recalled dancing until three in the morning and screaming with laughter at stories of the guys' college days. If this was to be the last of these parties, it would certainly be unforgettable. But, Kate smiled to herself, George would probably find a way to make it back for future parties. Feeling drained from all the emotion, Kate suppressed a yawn.

"Okay," announced Sam, standing up and poking Kate in the stomach to interrupt her yawn. "I'd better be going. It's late for a work night." He left, promising Matt a game of tennis for the following evening.

As Kate shut the door behind him, she silently prayed Matt would not bring up the emotional scene that had taken place before Sam's visit. She busied herself with the empty glasses and coffee cups.

"You don't have to tell me about it," said Matt, as he helped her bring the cups into the kitchen. "But I am concerned about you. You're my pal."

Tempted as she was to pour her heart out to him, she said simply, "It's nothing, really. And it is so late. You must be tired."

"I don't believe you that it's nothing, Kate Bennett," Matt countered, standing with his hands on his hips and blocking her path. "I am not too tired to listen to you. I *care* about you. It is never good to leave these things unresolved."

"Oh, God," Kate began. Matt guided her to the nearest kitchen chair and sat down across from her. She took a deep breath and launched into the story that she knew could ruin any chance she and Matt might have. "I told you I was married, right? Well, it was no picnic. Of course not; if it had been good, I would probably still be married and back in New York," she said with a little laugh.

She looked up and saw him leaning over the table, encouraging her with his eyes to go on. "I don't know when things started to go wrong," she continued, "but I know I didn't recognize Mitch's alcohol problem when we first met. Christ, I was so blinded by infatuation…"

Kate felt the story unravelling practically on its own, and it seemed like a movie she had seen several months ago that had grown fuzzy in her memory. After all, she had confided in several others before this: Jackie, her therapist, Sam. She no longer felt the same emotional attachment to the story, almost as if it had happened to somebody else. When she got to the part about Mitch's throwing the dishes on the floor and kicking a hole in the door, she stopped to recall the details.

Matt interpreted this pause as emotional and took her hand in his. When she told him that Mitch had never hit her, Matt said, "Thank God", sighing profoundly with relief. "I don't want to imagine anyone hurting you physically."

This touched her to the core and she suddenly felt embarrassed, as though she had no right to involve Matt in her personal heartache. She racked her brain for a way to continue. "Oh, Matt. I've been so wary of most men since then. Meeting someone as genuine and caring as you…I don't know how to deal with it."

"It's all right, Kate." His voice was so gentle, smoothed away all the rough edges around her fragile emotions.

It should have been so simple. It had felt simple on the couch, the passion carrying them away like the strong winds of the Sahara. But as they reached the vortex of the great whirlwind, it was all silent and deathly still. Without the wind whipping at her, she did not know which way to turn. "Matt, I don't know what it is I feel for you, I mean, obviously I'm attracted to you, but I wouldn't want anything to jeopardize our friendship..."

Matt responded by squeezing her hand which was still in his. "I'm glad you told me about your past. Now, let's concentrate on the future, which starts tomorrow morning, bright and early." He stood and faced her. "Are you okay?" His look conveyed such an earnest concern that she had to smile.

"Of course, I'm okay. Thanks for being patient with me."

He just grinned and let himself out the front door, after giving Kate a kiss on the cheek.

Something felt unresolved. Kate went over the conversation again in her head and smiled. He was so perfect. Anyone else would have been completely disgusted with her antics, she knew. On an impulse, she ran out the front door after Matt and caught up with him halfway between her place and his.

His look betrayed his amusement as she skidded to a stop before crashing into him. "I...I forgot to give you something," she gasped. She reached up and threw her arms around his neck to hug him tightly. "That's to say thanks." It felt so good to hug him that she clutched onto him even harder.

Moonlight blended with the lamplight in the car park to create a mysterious cast to their surroundings. Matt let Kate pull away gradually, although both were unconcerned about this kind of display. After all, it was the middle of the night and their neighbors were probably fast asleep. She sighed. "I suppose we'd better call it a night."

"I'd call it morning, actually," he remarked, showing her

the time on his watch. "I'll see you in about three hours." They both groaned and went their separate ways, Kate feeling lighter and happier than she had in months.

Chapter 6

"I found the granola bars!" Rita McGregor yelled across the health food store. She held up a handful of blue and red wrapped bars. "Do we want peanut or oat and honey?"

Kate came around the side of the display aisle. "You choose, Rita, but remember people have different preferences." It had been Kate's idea to plan a Healthy Halloween party, an attempt to celebrate the holiday in a more modern context that reflected the way people had started to live their lives. She and Matt had driven seven students to the health food store to choose some treats that were chemical- and preservative-free.

In Matt's car on the way, he had had one of the students read off the ingredients on a package of M&M's before tearing open the bag and doling out the colorful candies. "One last ceremonial sacrifice," he had said, with a twinkle in his eye. "Don't tell Miss Bennett."

They headed back to the school with the ingredients for Kate's "different kind of Halloween". When they arrived at Ramon, there was only one half hour before the festivities were due to commence, and Kate hurriedly assigned jobs to the students. She sent Pedro Morales with Matt to get the Halloween decorations and costumes from the basement.

Matt had suggested the gym for the party's venue, and

Kate had agreed it was the only room big enough to hold everyone. About half of the staff had decided to join in, along with their students. There were several bags of fruit and nuts lined up against the equipment cages, and Kate started putting the contents onto the enormous trays borrowed from the cafeteria.

Pedro suddenly came running back into the gym, screaming, "Miss Bennett, Miss Bennett, come quick!" He waved both arms in a frantic gesture, and tugged on Kate's arm to lead her.

"What's happened, Pedro?" she asked in a trembling voice, fearing the worst. She quickened her pace as she followed him to the basement.

Pedro recounted the incident in his broken English which seemed to have worsened from the fear. Apparently, Matt had gone to turn on the basement light, but had slipped on a loose tile and fallen head first down the entire flight of stairs. As Kate reached for the light, she found the bulb had blown, and she slowly made her way down the stairs in the dark.

Matt was lying on the basement floor, with his feet still on the stairs, and as Kate's eyes became accustomed to the dark, she could see that he was unconscious, but his legs were twitching in unevenly spaced, jerky movements.

"Pedro!" she called, amazed that she could get any sound out, "Go get Mr. Price. Tell him what happened, and ask him to call an ambulance and come down here. You, return to the gym, and please don't say anything to the other students yet." She looked up the stairs, saw him nod and run off.

Alone with Matt, Kate reached out to touch him, but decided against it. She saw a small stain near his head and touched it. Sticky. Blood. She began to cry and prayed for Eddie to hurry up. Matt's body was convulsing, first short jerks, then longer ones, and Kate moved to sit a few steps up, heartbroken and horrified. There was a brief period of quiet, and Kate leaned over Matt's still body, terrified. He began another convulsion just as Eddie came pounding down the stairs.

Thankful for his presence and that of Mary Sinclair, whom Eddie had brought with him, Kate tried her best to explain what had happened. Mary went over and put her arm around Kate's shoulders, murmuring soothing words. Eddie went upstairs to show the paramedics to the scene of the accident.

When Mary offered to take over the running of the Halloween party, Kate instantly agreed, not wanting to leave Matt's side, in case he woke up disoriented. She accompanied him into the ambulance, sitting as close to him as the bulky medical equipment would allow. One of the paramedics also sat in the back of the vehicle, trying to hold an oxygen mask to Matt's face. Suffering through another two convulsions, Matt knocked the oxygen mask off and a flailing arm unconsciously hit the paramedic in the face.

Kate felt her hot tears burning her eyes and cheeks as they kept falling in an endless curtain. She waved away the paramedic's offer of a paper bag to breathe into, willing herself to stop hyperventilating so she could be of more help. But, watching Matt in his silent agony, she knew she could not go near him because he was not in control of his violent movements. She shrank back and crouched helplessly in the corner of the ambulance, praying.

"Miss Bennett." The shrill voice reached through the film of unreality, and Kate looked into the face of a young female doctor. "I'm sorry to bother you again," the doctor continued, "but we need you to confirm that Mr. Reynolds has no history of epilepsy, and that no one in his family does." Kate shook her head slowly, not wanting to talk any more. For an hour after Matt's admission to the hospital, Kate had been forced to answer questions and more questions about Matt's general health and medical history. She had excused herself after a short while, to call Matt's mother. Pulling herself together, she had carefully explained the incident to Mrs. Reynolds, assuring her that he was safe now. Mrs. Reynolds had assured her that nothing like this had ever happened before, and it made Kate feel responsible somehow, as though the accident would never have happened had Matt remained in Tucson.

Convincing herself that this was nonsense, she managed to give Mrs. Reynolds directions to the hospital, and tried to persuade her to wait until the next morning to set off in the car. No, she had sighed, he is not conscious yet. But he is in very good hands. She hoped that her voice conveyed more confidence than she felt. Matt's mother said she thought they would leave immediately for Scottsdale, and thank you very much, Kate, for taking care of everything. Kate cringed as she remembered the ride in the ambulance. Sure, no problem. See you soon. Drive safely.

A barrage of questions ensued when Kate returned to the nurses' station, able to confirm the details of Matt's health. It was so tiring; all she wanted to do was make sure Matt was all right.

"Thank you, Miss Bennett. You can see the patient for ten minutes, now, but he is still unconscious."

Kate went right up to Matt's bed and looked at him closely. She would have thought he was just sleeping if it were not for the tubes in his nose and the intravenous needle dripping some clear liquid into his arm. Noticing the straps tightly holding his wrists and ankles to the bed, Kate began to cry again. She was still hovering over his bed when a nurse arrived to ask her to leave. He would still be unconscious for another few hours, she was told. *How the hell do you know?* Kate thought angrily. *Do you really know what he is going through?* But there was no one for Kate to ask, and she left the hospital room, feeling as helpless as before, and defeated.

After puttering around the house for two hours, wandering aimlessly, she called Mary on the telephone to fill her in on the hospital ordeal. She listened to Mary's low voice reassuring her that they had done all the right things, and felt somewhat comforted. She then called Jackie in Denver. Ever since Jackie had moved there, the two women had made a real effort to stay in touch, through weekly phone calls and sporadic letters. Kate knew she could still count on Jackie to help her feel more like herself. She hung up the phone a half hour later, energy restored and spirit uplifted.

She practically jumped into her car to return to the hospital.

Walking down the corridor toward Matt's room, Kate could see a young girl's back through the door which was ajar. She slowed her footsteps as she reached the door. Kate knew in an instant that Matt's mother had arrived from Tucson with one of her daughters. She tapped lightly on the door to announce her arrival, and Matt's mother looked up, still kneeling by Matt's bed and fingering a rosary.

"Hello, Mrs. Reynolds." Kate's voice was a whisper, betraying the frailness she felt as a result of the situation.

Matt's mother stood and went over to Kate with a warm smile. The two women hugged each other, breaching the gap in age, background, and experience with a blanket of comfort and shared sorrow. They sat in the two plastic chairs that were meant for visitors and Kate told the story of the accident, this time in more detail. She paused several times for Mrs. Reynolds to wipe her eyes and blow her nose, and she soon found herself forgetting her own sorrow to comfort the woman who had given birth to her newest yet almost closest friend.

When Matt had not awakened by nine o'clock that evening, Kate went to talk to the nurses to see if she could find out anything else. They shook their heads and pointed her in the direction of the young doctor.

"It's hard to tell," hedged Doctor Anderson. "We have given him five hundred milligrams of phenytoin to stabilize him. He may sleep straight through till tomorrow morning." She looked at Kate openly and shrugged. "Maybe you should go home and rest. You've had quite an ordeal yourself."

Kate tried hard not to resent this young representative of the medical profession. She knew from some of her college friends that had gone on to medical school how difficult it was to diagnose accurately. Nevertheless, she still felt so out of control, as if someone else had decided to direct her life without telling her. She knew she was looking for a shred of comfort from this young doctor, even if it was a guess; then, she could go home knowing that Matt would probably be better tomorrow.

Dr. Anderson joined Kate and Mrs. Reynolds for a cup of coffee in one of the waiting areas, since the cafeteria had closed for the night. "I know I can't feel what you're feeling," the doctor stated plainly, "but I do have experience with this type of accident, and the prognosis is excellent." She nodded confidently, looking from Mrs. Reynolds to Kate for support.

Matt's mother spoke first. "Matt has been through many challenges in his short life. I have no doubt he will come through this just fine."

Kate grasped onto this statement since it held more weight for her than a stranger's view, albeit a medical one. She wanted the faith of this religious woman to carry them all to safety.

Suddenly, Kate was overwhelmed by the exhaustion of the day, and realized that the doctor was probably right in sending them home. After one last look at Matt's sleeping form, Kate managed to get Mrs. Reynolds to follow her back to Sunny Vista. They woke Matt's sister Sarah, who had fallen asleep in one of the leather chairs in the waiting area, and drove slowly to the development.

After getting the Reynolds settled in Matt's house, Kate went home and collapsed into bed. She awoke with a start to the jarring sound of the phone. It was Alan Coon, principal at Ramon.

"Hello, Kate," he boomed over the telephone line. "I know you will probably not be coming in today, so don't worry, we've got a substitute lined up." Kate glanced over to her clock and was shocked to see that it was already eight-fifteen in the morning. She groaned inwardly as Alan continued, "I was really just calling to see how Matt is doing."

She sighed and told him what had happened the previous day, promising to keep him updated since she was heading to the hospital very soon.

"I am very concerned about him, Kate. Please let me know when he is well enough for visitors." Kate could hear the anxiety in Coon's voice, but something about it did not sound genuine. She agreed to let him know anyway and mulled over Coon's comments once more before dozing for another few hours.

"Matt!" Kate screamed with delight to see him sitting almost upright in the bed, watching television. She wanted to hug him, but was deterred by the tangle of tubes and sheets. Instead, she kissed him lightly on his cheek, trying to aim for a spot with no bruises.

He flinched slightly anyway. "Oh, Kate," he said with a wry smile, "I feel like somebody put my whole body through a meat grinder." He rolled his eyes for effect and Kate laughed. He told her how when he woke up, he tried to get up to go to the bathroom, and found his arms and legs strapped to the bed. "So, I just yelled and the nurses came running. I laughed to see them running in here so fast just to help me take a piss, but I don't think they thought it was very funny. Ow, ow, it hurts." He tried to stop laughing, which was obviously hurting his bruised body, but the more he tried to stop, the more he laughed, and Kate soon joined in.

Matt's mother came into the room with a small basket of flowers that had just arrived. It was from the staff at Ramon, wishing Matt a speedy recovery. Mrs. Reynolds placed the flowers on a table near the window then went over to stroke Matt's head. "I was so worried about you," she said with a long sigh. "But Kate took good care of you until I got here, didn't she?" She put her hand on Kate's shoulder and beamed at her gratefully.

"Yeah, Kate's my buddy." Matt lifted his hand carefully and touched Kate's. "Thanks," he said quietly, and the soft tone made Kate feel a bit uncomfortable. *After all*, she thought, *I didn't really do anything. I just stood there.* She shook her head almost imperceptibly.

She resolved mentally to stay with Matt as much as she could until he got better. He remained in good spirits for most of the day, tiring only after his medication every four hours. Kate was able to take a few more days off to be with Matt and she watched him improve slowly. She was reading a magazine during one of Matt's naps when Eddie, Mary, and two other teachers came in.

"Shh!" Kate put her finger to her lips and pointed to Matt, who was snoring softly. She went out to join them for a cup of coffee. They told her how Alan Coon had pressed them for details about the accident and then surveyed the basement stairs like a detective. Eddie had commented that the light bulb had blown, and Coon had practically snapped his head off with his retort.

"Apparently," said Mary, knowingly, "he's particularly worried about the school's liability in this. He can't hide the fact that there was a burnt out light bulb and a loose tile, though. Matt could have killed himself!" She said this last sentence in a tone of wonder, as though she had only just realized the severity of the situation.

Reliving the horror of that day, when she groped her way in the darkness toward Matt's unconscious form, Kate shuddered. She let the reality of it permeate her mind once again. It was all very well for Mary to make her comments, but she had not witnessed Matt's pain when the accident actually occurred. Well, neither had Kate, come to think of it. By the time she reached Matt, the major convulsions had ceased. None of them could really say what Matt had experienced.

Oh, Matt, I'm sorry, Kate thought miserably. *If only I had gone to get the costumes myself. If only you hadn't been in such a rush. If only the light bulb had been working. If only...*but it really did no good to dwell on it.

"Sssh!" Eddie Price tried to get the other teachers to lower their voices, which had risen gradually in excited talk and jokes. He cast a suspicious eye at Matt, who was still sleeping peacefully. "Maybe we should hang out in the lounge or something, you know. We don't want to wake Sleeping Beauty." Nobody seemed to want to make a move. It was as though even in repose Matt asserted a sort of leadership over them, and as long as he was in the room, the rest of them gathered around him in a loose circle of admiration.

So the group of teachers stayed in Matt's room, talking and joking. Matt remained asleep the whole time, although the slight smile on his lips made Kate think he was possibly faking, waiting to hear what everyone had to say about him. Kate wondered if she should say something shocking to test him, but decided that was too mean. A loud snore told her he was truly asleep. *Nobody could fake that noise*, Kate thought and almost giggled out loud.

At about six o'clock that evening, the nurse alerted them that visiting hours had ended. Kate did not want the comfort of companionship to end, so she invited the whole group to her place for dinner. She couldn't remember how clean the kitchen had been when she left, but she could always clean up quickly.

When they got in, Mary took over in the kitchen, giving orders to the other four to prepare an impromptu feast from the contents of Kate's cupboards. Her cool manner was the perfect balance between authoritative and controlled. "Give me that tomato paste, Eddie. And that large spoon over there."

"Yes, sir," Eddie responded with a smirk, following her instructions. The other teachers were stacking pots and pans for washing, and clearing the table to make room for place settings.

Kate watched the scene in mild amusement; she was glad the group could make themselves at home in her house. And Mary obviously had dinner under control.

Sensing that she was not really needed, Kate collapsed into the soft couch and relaxed for the first time in a week. It occurred to her that she had not thought about anything but Matt's condition for that whole time. The idea made her happy: she was finally being the kind of friend she had always wanted to be.

Chapter 7

Matt picked up the book and flicked through it swiftly, stopping to read some key section and nodding excitedly. "Yes, this is very good," he commented. "It gets right to the heart of the matter and gives you practical ideas for overcoming the distractions." Ever since Matt had told Kate about meditation, she had been intrigued, but it was not until he extolled its virtues for eliminating his constant pain that she finally went to the local library to take out some books on the subject. Now, she was asking Matt to judge the quality of the books, since he had warned her about the plethora of obtuse and inaccurate sources in print.

"Tell me again what you want me to do," she reminded him now, fearful of "getting it wrong" and doing some serious harm to her body or mind.

Matt handed her the book. "I think this is a good one. But you'll have to judge that for yourself. The one thing you should do is read it slowly and carefully, not at your normal rabbit pace. Stop after every chapter and try to do the things he suggests."

"I don't know..." Kate looked doubtful. She was genuinely frightened of embarking on the subject of meditation on her own because she thought her overactive mind was ill-suited to the task. Maybe I could meditate with you," she offered in a small voice.

"Sure, why not?" Matt seemed agreeable. He meditated every day in the hospital room, shutting out the noise of the carts squeaking down the corridors and the pain afflicting his healing body. Kate had only seen him doing it once, and when he had heard her enter the room, he had opened his eyes and smiled at her. When Kate had pressed him for more of an explanation about it, he had elaborated with fascinating stories of Zen teachers and students in Japan and their ability to transcend the everyday annoyances of life.

Kate felt like jumping up and down when Matt explained it this way, since it described so perfectly her life and her tendency to let things drive her crazy, causing frequent headaches and anxiety. Matt had mentioned more than once that it may take Kate a while to master the seemingly simple sitting meditation, but the aura of mystique about the whole practice was stronger than any apprehensions she had about the challenge. Yes, she definitely wanted to try this exercise that had apparently helped others achieve such a calm and stable state of mind.

"We could start tomorrow morning," Matt suggested, happy for the opportunity to teach again, since he had been away from the school for a week and a half.

"I have to go to work," Kate reminded him with a gentle jab to his arm. "But, definitely Saturday. And you might even be home by then. That would be good." Kate knew how much Matt detested being in the hospital, helpless and bored, and having to contend with the patronizing doctors day after day. He had won most of the staff over with his sense of humor and charm, but Kate suspected it might be starting to wear thin.

They agreed to start the meditation lessons on Saturday, whether Matt was at home or still in the hospital. Kate's assignment was to read the first chapter of the meditation book and to pick out the ideas that appealed to her.

"And you're not going to expect miracles, right, Bennett?" Matt laughed. "Because I've never taught anyone meditation before."

She shook her head. No miracles. But there was a certain thrill of anticipation that something fantastic was about to begin.

As she drove home, she reflected on the idea of meditating. Never would she have been so excited back in New York about sitting quietly and doing nothing. Quite the opposite, in fact; it would have frustrated her no end to have to remain still and let all of her distracting thoughts float away. She smiled to herself, glad that Matt had agreed to help her get started.

Saturday morning was ushered in by a quick early-morning storm, which dissipated around ten o'clock, just when Kate was getting into her car to drive down to the hospital. Dr. Anderson and her colleagues had agreed that Matt could go home, as long as he took his medication regularly and showed up for weekly visits to check the condition. All of the doctors were too vague for Kate's exacting mind, and they failed to answer the question about whether Matt had developed epilepsy when he fell down the stairs, or whether he merely suffered some severe convulsions from the impact, and would never be bothered again.

But, as Matt bounced into the passenger seat, after kissing the nurses goodbye and shaking hands with the doctors that had assembled to see him off, Kate forgot about everything except having her friend back. She had tried to keep him up to date on the events back at Ramon, so he wouldn't feel too lonely and alienated, and they chatted about the school for the duration of the drive home.

When they reached Matt's apartment, Kate was surprised to hear him say that he wanted a short nap and then they would meditate. She had almost forgotten that they had agreed to start this morning. She nodded absentmindedly, her thoughts already filled with the thrill of beginning something new, but shaky at the same time, like a child about to board an airplane for the first time. She desperately wanted to learn to meditate, although she realized that her excitement itself was probably going to be a big distraction. Matt had explained this to her.

They sat cross-legged on the carpet in Matt's living room, having dimmed the sunlight by closing the curtains. Kate was still impressed by the thorough nature of Arizona residents when it came to adjusting the climate to suit their comfort. The air conditioning felt cool against their slightly sweaty skin.

Matt began in a quiet voice, walking Kate through an exercise to relax her body, limb by limb. He had her focus on each part of the body as he coached her to let go of the tightness and anxiety of the week. Kate kept her eyes closed and her mind started to focus on her breathing. When Matt announced that the session was over, Kate opened her eyes and was stunned to see that nearly an hour had passed.

"That was amazing!" she said, breathlessly. She thought her concentration could have been better, though, since she had had many thoughts enter her mind, distracting her, but Matt said that was normal.

"It will take time," he nodded knowingly. "If you stick with it, though, you will really notice a difference. My first time was a total disaster. There was this rooster who kept crowing and every time my mind wandered to follow its shrill call, my Zen master poked me with a bamboo cane. I don't know how he knew my thoughts were on that rooster..." Matt shook his head in amazement, his gaze very far away for a moment.

"Well!" he was back now. "How about some tea? "

Kate stretched out on the carpet while Matt made the tea. She observed the sparse furnishings and decorations that her friend had chosen and decided that they reflected his taste perfectly. Matt would never accumulate clutter the way most of the other men Kate knew would. He preferred the simple arrangement of an empty vase next to another small vase containing a single tiger lily; abhorring ostentatiousness of any kind, was he perhaps making a statement?

Kate was pondering this last thought when she heard the sound of a teacup smashing against ceramic tiles. "What are you doing?" she teased. "Can't I trust you to make a simple cup of tea?" She wandered into the kitchen, where Matt was standing, dumbstruck, looking at the pieces of cup scattered across the floor.

He shook his head slowly. "It's the craziest thing, Kate. I just watched as my hand began to tremble and then it was impossible to hold the cup.

Like a small seizure, but just my hand." He continued to shake his head in disbelief.

"Are you okay?" she asked, her eyes wide with worry.

Matt nodded. "Yeah, it lasted for about fifteen seconds, then it was over. Just like that." He was staring at his hand, amazed at the whole occurrence. Curling and uncurling his fingers, he added, "There's just a vague tingling sensation to remind me."

After ensuring that he was feeling better, Kate picked up a newspaper and swept the broken pieces together to throw out. Matt got out another cup and continued pouring the tea as if nothing had happened. She said she thought maybe he should call Dr. Anderson.

"Come on," he snarled, angrier than Kate would have expected. Then he smiled, the fierce look replaced by a playful one. "It's nothing. And, furthermore, it's over. I'll tell her about it when I see her on Tuesday." He said this to appease Kate, who had taken to mothering him slightly ever since the accident.

They took their tea into the living room and relaxed on the soft sea of beige that covered most of the living room floors at Sunny Vista. Kate was surprised when Matt asked if her students were behaving any better. She hadn't realized that she had mentioned any of her frustrations to him.

"They just don't seem to have any respect for education, and certainly not for the teachers. Well, not all of them are like that," she added, not wanting to sound completely intolerant. She was actually fairly proud of her progress in terms of getting the students to take responsibility for their belongings and their behavior in her classroom. She shuddered to think of what happened outside the classroom.

"I don't see that they are any worse than your average, hormone-stricken, confused adolescents. Come on, Kate, don't you remember when you were their age? It wasn't all that long ago." Matt always tried to shorten the age gap between the young teachers and the students, while Kate tried to widen it. The friendly companionship that he appeared to have with his students was not something she wanted, nor did she deem it appropriate. She felt strongly that there should be a sense of authority, otherwise, what is to prevent the students from making all their own rules? She bit her lip, feeling that any argument would only push them further apart on this issue.

Matt sipped his tea thoughtfully. Kate knew that he was deciding whether to push her on this or not, and she felt like laughing out loud, imagining him picturing a wild-eyed, violent scene from her. He jumped up suddenly and picked up their empty teacups. "I'll tell you what," he said. "Let's take some of the students out to dinner next week. You know, a kind of field trip. You can choose your kids any way you want. Okay?"

"Oh, I don't know. Do you really want to deal with them at a restaurant, of all places? You know how they can act in the cafeteria." She was not at all sure she like this idea of his.

He waved her scepticism away with his hand. "That's why I said you can pick your students any way you want. I'm sure there are *some* that deserve to go." He paused deliberately to let the words sink in. Kate marvelled at Matt's ability to turn the situation around. A dinner out with her students, now *that* was something new. Sure, why not?

C. Ramon Junior High School looked more imposing somehow as Kate's car turned into the drive. To Matt's dismay, Dr. Anderson had prohibited him from driving until "further notice", which basically meant until there was no danger of having a seizure behind the wheel. When he had pressed her for a more precise answer, she had told him that two years completely seizure-free was the common rule. Oh, my God. He was thankful that Kate lived so close, and of course she had offered to take him to the school and back home each day. It had only been two weeks since the accident, but it felt like much longer to Matt, who had been growing impatient to return to work.

As they entered the great front hall, students and teachers alike crowded around him to hear his side of the story; some of the tales that had become exaggerated by young imaginative minds included such details as Matt's head splitting in two and his face turning into that of a monster. But, he seemed to be his cheerful self, and there was virtually no physical evidence left of the accident, except for a faint bruise on his left temple.

Smiling to herself, Kate took her books and papers up to the classroom. *He's in his element*, she told herself. Storyteller par excellence with a flair for the dramatic. She wondered if his version of the story would become even more fantastic than those imagined by the students.

The glass of beer shone like gold in the late afternoon sunlight. It had been Kate's idea to go to Shorty's for a drink before meeting the students at the restaurant, and as she felt the warm glow overpower the fatigue that had built up during the week, she was glad she had thought of it. She held up the glass to get the reflection to land on the table. It looked so refreshing, she couldn't wait to have a sip. Then she noticed Matt staring at her with an exaggerated pout on his face.

"Oh, I'm sorry," she said as she put the glass down. Dr. Anderson had prohibited Matt from drinking anything alcoholic, until the effects of the drugs were established. Never much of a drinker, the inaccessibility of it made Matt suddenly want a drink even more. Kate gulped down the remaining beer in her glass as if to hide the evidence.

"No, don't worry about me," he moaned. "I'll just enjoy my *orange juice*." He spat out the words with distaste. "Just think how much healthier I'll be than you, my health food freak." He thought it was very amusing that Kate lectured her friends about eating right and exercising, then drank whatever she wanted when they went out.

"I go running or swim a few times a week, I eat salad just about every day. I say that gives me the right to indulge now and then."

Matt looked at her, unconvinced.

"Alcohol is good for you, in small quantities. Well, good for *me* anyway." The more she tried not to remind him of a drink, the harder it seemed not to mention it.

"You've always taken care of your body, too, haven't you?" she asked, changing the subject. She caressed his leg under the table with her foot. Waited to see if he would rise to the bait.

One long steady look later, Matt downed his orange juice. "I do my best. Yeah," he admitted, "I do take some pride in my body. It's important."

There was a thrill as Kate contemplated following through with this line of thought. She could feel the solid line of his leg next to hers. The heat emanating from it was exciting, but at the same time familiar. She almost longed to touch him, right now, right here in Shorty's, and to hell with the faculty gossip that would surely ensue. She pressed her leg against Matt's a bit harder now, pressing her luck with it. She kept her gaze steady on Matt's amber eyes.

But it was nearly five-thirty, the designated meeting time for dinner. "Let's get going," she prompted, pulling her self-control into action and rising from her chair.

Japanese music drifted into the room which was decorated in what Kate assumed was a very traditional manner. Paper lanterns of various colors moved gently as they hung from the ceiling, casting a soft light on the other people dining in the restaurant. The effect was almost surreal.

The eight students led the way to a long table set for the large group. Kate looked around the young faces and felt grateful to Matt for organizing this outing which would help them to get to know some students a little better. She had chosen the four top students for the week, brandishing the dinner as a prize. Matt had invited four of the students that he worked with on an individual basis.

Matt wasted no time in calling over one of the waiters, whom he had apparently met on a previous visit to the restaurant. Listening to him order exotic dishes in Japanese, most of the table fell silent, except for two or three students trying to imitate the strange syllables.

"You all like fish eyes, right?" Matt joked. "Just to remind you that he who can order in Japanese is in charge." After assuring some of the girls who were close to tears that he was teasing, he began to delight them with stories of his adventures in Japan.

The meal passed quickly, with delicious dishes complementing the lively events Matt was describing. At one point, she leaned over to ask him in a whisper if he was telling the truth, and he raised his eyebrows in mock horror.

"Of course, my dear Kate," was all he said, and she decided that it didn't really matter anyway. She glanced at the young faces mesmerized by Matt's charm and smiled to herself. *They're hooked,* she thought. *They've all got crushes on Matt Reynolds. No, not they, but rather we have all got crushes on this magical person. But,* Kate reassured herself, *I've got mine under control.*

Suddenly, Matt snapped his head around, something behind the sushi bar having caught his eye. "Look," he whispered. When the group followed his pointing finger to the wall behind the bar, they observed a long, curved sword with an intricately carved silver hilt.

"That's a Samurai sword," Matt explained, never taking his eye off the object. "If it's authentic, then it's at least four hundred years old." He beckoned to one of the waiters and spoke a few words to him in Japanese.

"Hai, so desu." The waiter nodded his head vigorously as he replied. It's true.

"Well, is it, Mr. Reynolds?" Tim Peterson could not contain his curiosity.

Matt looked Tim squarely in the eye. "That sword," he began in a voice hushed with reverence, "belonged to a Samurai warrior in the sixteenth century. It has been handed down in the owner's family, all the way from his great-great-great-great-grandfather, or something. "

Tim laughed.

"That sword contains magic," Matt admonished him with a penetrating look. Just think of the warrior that possessed that magical instrument of death, flying at his opponent in a flash of powerful action. Unhesitating, unafraid, the warrior advances. Then, with a mighty shout rising up from the depths of his soul, he leaps." There was a hushed silence around the table, vibrating with anticipation of the end of the story.

Finally drawing his attention away from the sword and back to the table, Matt put a piece of sushi in his mouth and savored its subtle, succulent taste.

"Well, what happened Mr. Reynolds?"

"Yeah, what happened?"

Kids. Matt snickered to himself. "What do you mean, what happened? I just told you what happened."

"But did he die, the warrior?" This came from one of the girls, the worried look in her eyes nearly as strong as her desire to hear the details of the gory battle.

"Yes, Susan, he died. But in Japan," Matt explained, "it's not a question of dying or not dying. The noble Samurai warrior was trained to fight his hardest in battle, yet to be prepared for his own death as much as his opponent's. He would not have been afraid to die, if he died in battle, the honorable way."

"I've seen them movies," Tim piped up. (Kate fought back the urge to correct his grammar). "You know, with the Kamikaze fighter pilots? Man, they looked so cool, flying their planes right at their targets and then, Boom! That's when the plane blew up and the guy inside was fried, you know he was." Tim nodded his head excitedly at the rest of the students who had turned their attention to him.

Aware that Tim had captured their respect, Matt confirmed the boy's story. "The Kamikaze can be seen as the modern-day Samurai. I know it may be hard for you all to believe, but the glory of dying in action is so attractive to those warriors that they rushed to sign up during World War II. You're right, Tim, it is a beautiful thing to watch, a man putting his honor above everything else."

So simple, he made it seem. Kate admired the way he held the kids in rapture with further stories of the Samurai and their adventures. One of the boys wanted to touch the sword, but the proprietor was wary of taking it down from the wall.

"If we leave it where it is," Matt compromised, "the magic will stay in the sword itself. If we took it down, something bad might happen to it and some of the magic would be lost."

Something bad might happen, Kate chuckled inwardly. *Yeah, like one of them might cut himself.* She was glad the sword was staying on the wall. The students appeared content with Matt's answer. Kate just hoped they could move the conversation away from the gruesome and onto something more pleasant. She asked Matt to tell them about the cherry blossom festival in the springtime.

A shower of *sayonaras* and *domo arigatos* escorted the group out the door, and they shouted back, eager to use the foreign words that evoked such wonderful fantasies. Silently, she thanked Matt for making it happen: for suggesting it, for planning it, for entertaining the kids with his stories. More than ever, she desired to visit Japan, especially with Matt as a tour guide.

Diligent parents had all arrived to pick their children up. One by one, the students tugged on Matt's arm to introduce him to their parents. It didn't seem to matter that they were in the middle of a restaurant parking lot and the evening was getting late. They dragged him from car to car as though he were a politician shaking hands and kissing babies.

What a great effect he has on them, Kate thought to herself, once they had finally said all their goodbyes and were heading home in the car. She hoped she could be that good with the kids. She would aspire to be that good.

Chapter 8

Over the past couple of weeks, Kate had seen Sam several times, first telling him the news about Matt's accident, then going together with him to visit Matt in the hospital. They had spent a rather uncomfortable evening together last week, Kate imagining that Sam's circumspect glances at her hid something deeper, that he was reluctant to divulge. Toward the end of the evening, Kate felt that they were getting closer to the way they had been in the past, but there was no way to span the awkward silences that plagued their conversation.

Unwilling to let things fester any longer, Kate had invited Sam to an outdoor concert on the field of the town hall. They reclined on an old blanket that Sam used for such occasions and drank wine out of paper cups. When Kate broached the subject of their friendship, she thought she saw a flicker of appreciation in Sam's dark eyes.

"I'm sorry we haven't had much time for each other lately," he began tentatively. Observing Kate's downcast eyes, he continued, "I really miss the old days. I miss George like you would not believe."

Hearing this from Sam's lips made Kate feel more selfish and foolish for not having recognized it before. She rubbed Sam's shoulder affectionately and wondered if he wanted her to say something. Searching for the words, she found none that could explain how her friendship with Matt had taken over her life. It was probably obvious to Sam, who had also become friendly with Matt, but, she imagined, not in the same way; rather, in a "guys" kind of way. *Surely, he must know what a magnetic personality Matt can be,* she rationalized, *but that has just made our ill-fated union more impossible than ever.* She felt her stomach turn over in anticipation of the sincere talk she had been wanting to have with Sam for about a year.

"You love him, don't you?" Sam's face was open and his expression kind.

Kate felt catapulted into a torrent of emotional winds. Sam had stated it so easily, nonchalantly, but there was nothing easy or nonchalant about the way she was feeling. Her head felt light as she weighed the question, incredulous. She *couldn't* love Matt. She honestly didn't think she did, but Sam had gotten that idea from somewhere. She shook her head. "It's not like that, Sam." It sounded so lame, and Kate wished, not for the first time, that she had a scriptwriter for these instances.

"I understand," he said warmly. "It doesn't change the way I feel about you, or about Matt. I want us to all be friends." There was an underlying current of desperation as he spoke the words, implying that if things did not work out this way, he would have lost all of his close friends in a very short time.

It was too coincidental that ever since Kate had started to spend a lot of time with Matt, she had no time for Sam. And he had had to say goodbye to his best friend earlier that same year. He had known it would be different without George around, but he had not anticipated how empty the house would feel without his boisterous outbursts and attacks of mischievous playfulness. Sam had already realized that he must have taken

George's presence for granted, so long had they been living in the same house and sharing so many fun-filled moments.

Shifting uncomfortably on the blanket, Kate knew she could let the conversation drop or carry it through to its conclusion. She forced herself to answer Sam. "You are just as responsible for any lapse, you know. You may try and put all of the blame on me, but if you had been more assertive instead of sulking about it, you could have created more of an opportunity for us to see each other."

"You're absolutely right." She had not expected him to say this. "I have been so moody over the past few months that I haven't even seen fit to call you to see how you are doing." His dark eyes looked upward. "If I knew how to get out of those moods on my own, I would. It seems like a vicious circle, though. When you really need someone around, you can't seem to make a move towards them, it's like you're paralyzed by the sadness, by the self-pity. And they interpret that as your unwillingness to relate, so they leave you alone." Seeing the hurt look in Kate's eyes, Sam immediately put his arm around her.

"I don't mean you, necessarily. It's been happening with everyone lately. I feel so out of touch, as though the rug has been pulled out from under me. And until tonight, I haven't felt ready to take the first step out of this swampland of self-pity." He gazed at her gratefully. "But I hope you know I don't want anything from you, just your friendship and companionship."

"Of course." There wasn't a moment's hesitation. Kate felt grateful to Sam, also, for allowing her to feel needed. She still felt indebted to him, as though their relationship had been mostly one-sided in the past. But what about Sam's comment about Matt? Didn't that come from some sort of envy?

Against the backdrop of a particularly stunning piece of music, Kate poured some more wine into their paper cups. She tasted it, feeling it warm the back of her throat luxuriously. "What I worry more about," she continued, "is Matt's well-being. He had some kind of small seizure in his hand the other day that made him drop a teacup. I hope he really is okay, and not just playing it all down, the way he can."

At the mention of something medical, Sam's ears pricked up immediately. "What kind of small seizure?"

She shook her head. "I don't know what you call it. He just said his hand locked into a grip and a big spasm went through it. It was enough to drop the cup.

Sam ran his fingers through his dark hair. "Hmm," he stated ruminously. He didn't know too much about these things, but he found them fascinating. Always had.

"Is that the first time that's happened?"

"I don't know, Sam." Already, Kate was feeling guilty for discussing the coffee cup episode with Sam. She didn't feel right talking about Matt behind his back and told Sam this.

"Fine," he agreed good-naturedly. He stretched out on the blanket and breathed in the fresh night air. "Anyway," he said, after a few minutes, "I hope you understand what I was trying to tell you before. I don't mean to be antisocial. I need you around, it's just that I can't always bring myself to ask."

Comforted by his honesty, Kate leaned against Sam to listen to the last few strains of the music. They remained there, each lost in his thoughts while all around them, people folded up chairs and blankets, shouting goodbyes to each other and dragging small, sleepy children by the hand. Kate felt like she could stay like that forever: she was thankful that the problem had resolved itself, and she didn't want to touch the purity of the moment.

The next night, Sam, Matt, and Kate were sitting around the dining room table at Kate's place, relaxing after one of Kate's filling pasta dinners. Sam observed as Matt took out a small box from his shirt pocket, extracted two tiny pills, and swallowed them, washing them down with a glass of water.

"What are those for, buddy?" he asked, the pharmacologist in him genuinely interested.

Matt shrugged his shoulders. "I forget the name. I just call them my pink ones. Not to be confused with my little blue ones in the morning." He snapped the box shut and returned it to his breast pocket.

Dissatisfied with the answer, Sam dogged him, "But what are they supposed to do? Are they painkillers?"

Matt explained how Dr. Anderson, in collaboration with two other doctors, had determined that Matt would take the pills as a "precautionary measure", to ward off possible future seizures. The dosages were being monitored weekly, along with Matt's physiological reactions to the drugs.

"I don't understand," Sam pressed on. "Do you have epilepsy now, all of a sudden?" He had thought he understood what had happened when Matt fell down the stairs, and he had attributed the seizures to the impact of Matt's head hitting the basement stairs and floor so hard. But Matt had pretty much recovered from the incident, and Sam could not understand why his doctor was treating the case like that of an epilepsy patient.

Recounting the explanation that he had been given by Dr. Anderson, Matt described the monitoring and analysis in greater detail. He saw how his two friends were leaning over the table, intent on hearing every word, and he let out an explosive laugh. "My God, you guys, don't take everything so *seriously*!" he cried, waving the topic away with a big sweeping gesture. He jumped up, announcing that he had to feed his dog and that he would be right back.

When the door had closed behind him, Kate said quietly, "I'm still worried about him, Sam. He acts like it's nothing, but you know I told you about the other day, when his hand convulsed and he smashed a teacup? Matt told me earlier that he asked Dr. Anderson about it and it's called a focal seizure. Apparently, Matt could have these small seizures anytime, and there's no way to prepare for them." She sniffed. "He tells us not to be so serious. I don't think he's taking it seriously enough."

Sam patted her back, half patronizingly, half playfully. "What are you going to do about it, Kate Bennett? He's taking the medication. Leave it to the doctors who know more about this than you and I do." From his work in pharmaceuticals, Sam had developed a professional respect for doctors, who were, after all, his clients. He was impressed by their adventurous nature, demonstrated by their willingness to try new drugs on their patients in an effort to combat the particularly puzzling illnesses.

The sliding door opened and Kate started, expecting Matt to return via the front door. "This way was closer," he explained, "and I knew it would make Kate jump," he said to Sam in an aside.

Kate thought it would be extremely unfair to continue the discussion about Matt's medication, but she was shocked to hear the turn the conversation was taking.

It was Sam, in his "justice above all" mood, who asked Matt who was paying for the hospitalization and the follow-up treatment. Matt gave a noncommittal answer about the delays in the insurance claim forms, and Sam pounced.

"Why the hell don't you sue that stupid school? After all,

they were negligent about the basement light and the loose tiles. A prestigious institution like that would probably roll over immediately just to shut you up."

Matt shook his head. "I don't have it in for the school. To tell you the truth, I haven't decided if I'm going to pursue it at all. All I know is that if they had to come up with the kind of money that I think this costs, many programs at Ramon would suffer. I can't see doing that to the kids."

"You're an idiot!" Sam's nostrils were flaring as he shouted at his friend. Kate feared that he might hit Matt or even her in his rage. "Be smart, Reynolds. You can't pay for everything yourself. It's not fair!" He was pacing now, frustrated and determined to beat the system. Kate imagined him participating in such animated arguments on the Indian reservation, trying to see justice meted out to those who deserved it. Sam hit the back of a chair and continued pacing, now even more exasperated. "I just don't get it," he muttered. "Surely Ramon has some kind of insurance policy for accidents?" he tried hopefully.

Matt placed his hands on the table. "I haven't said I'm *not* suing the school," he conceded diplomatically. "I'm just torn, you see." And Kate was beginning to see; she hoped Sam was also. Matt's fierce loyalty was not to Ramon, but to the students to whom he was so devoted. The distress was evident in his face, grown pale and drawn over the past few weeks.

Meanwhile, Sam had stopped pacing. As he stood looking at one of Matt's prints on the wall, Kate watched his profile and saw the fluttery pulse of a nerve on his temple. She wondered if he was going to explode in another passionate outburst.

But he turned to them slowly and squatted down near Matt's chair, so he was almost at his level. "Do you want me to do anything for you?" he asked. "Research, or anything like that?" His tone had mellowed considerably. And he probably could find out a lot about different drugs at work.

"Thanks, buddy, but I can't think of anything." As Matt returned Sam's look, their eyes locked. "I will ask you to please stop acting like I'm an invalid, though. I'm fine, really." The discussion was over. Despite the smile, Kate could see the stress and worry underneath, but there was no mention of it now.

Later that night, as Kate was getting ready for bed, she went over the evening's conversation again in her head and realized that there had been no suitable answer to the question about financing Matt's medical expenses. She knew that his family could not afford to pay even the remainder of the crippling bills that had accumulated after ten days of hospitalization, continuous physical therapy, and medication.

Kate let her mind drift to Matt's mother, who had needed to return to Tucson after two days, amidst strenuous assurances from Kate as to Matt's welfare. She was definitely a strong woman, Frances Reynolds, and Kate could see what a positive role model she must have been. Matt had appreciated his mother's presence, as well as that of his little sister Sarah, but by the time they left, he had begun to assume a somewhat macho attitude, asserting his independence more fiercely than Kate had deemed necessary.

Kate lay awake, trying to fall asleep, but still alert and anxious about Matt and the financial burden that he was carrying in addition to the physical one. She thought about praying, but felt too out of touch with any God. Fighting back tears of anger and frustration, she got out of bed and went to the telephone.

"Hi, Jackie. Is it too late?"

The characteristic boisterous laugh. "It's never too late for you, Kate.

Even if it is two in the morning our time."

"Oh, God, I'm sorry. It's just that I really wanted to hear your voice." She proceeded to tell her friend about her frustrations. After all, she had not updated her except for another quick call to say Matt had regained consciousness. Now, as she tried to explain the situation, she realized how awful it must sound to someone who hadn't been part of it.

"Jesus, Kate." There was a sharp intake of breath, which Kate hoped was not a puff on a cigarette.

"He's perfectly fine now," Kate quickly defended Matt. "You wouldn't even know that anything had happened. But he's going to have to figure out how he can get the school to pay the bills without upsetting anybody too much."

"I know what hospital bills can be like."

For a second, Kate panicked, wondering if Jackie had been sick recently, but then she realized she must be speaking from professional experience.

"How's he handling it all?"

"Oh, you know Matt," Kate laughed. But, she realized, Jackie did not really know Matt at all, since she had left only a month after Matt had moved to town.

"He's the most incredible person, Jackie."

"Oh, yeah?" Jackie was intrigued. Despite all the experiences she and Kate had shared over the past ten years and all the men that had gone in and out of their lives, she couldn't remember ever hearing such a tone of admiration in Kate's voice.

The words couldn't come out fast enough as Kate tried to bring Jackie up to date on her friendship with Matt. She played it down, though, wouldn't admit there was anything more to it than a casual relationship.

"You're crazy," Jackie concluded. "If I were in your shoes, I would be all over him." She lowered her voice. "He saved my life that time, in the river."

"I thought so." There was a momentary pause as they both acknowledged this, Kate thanking Matt mentally, the admiration and wonder spilling over the surface once again. Indeed, Kate had forgotten about the incident in the river, had forgotten how clear of mind and quick to act Matt had been. And then, afterward, how humble, acting as though nothing had happened.

Talking to Jackie like this was just like old times; Kate could almost forget about the hundreds of miles between them. "Thanks for listening, Jackie." Yet again. "But it's very late, especially in Denver."

They said goodbye reluctantly, Kate promised to visit Jackie and George early in the new year. As she climbed into bed again, she felt a sense of exhaustion overtake her body and she knew she would be able to sleep.

Chapter 9

Alan Coon's desk gleamed in the fluorescent light of the small office; it betrayed one single smear, almost perfectly centered, from the dusting and polishing that it had received the day before. Matt sneered at the tidy little pile of papers placed at the upper righthand corner of the desk, wondering if Coon actually did any work. He caught himself thinking this way and was surprised at the antagonism he felt.

A moment later, Matt knew he was only reflecting the principal's own cold attitude back at him. He tried to focus his attention as Coon noisily scraped his chair into place, cleared his throat several times, and attempted, unsuccessfully, to make small talk.

"Matt, this is really just a chance for us to chat. I'd like to make sure that you are doing all right, both mentally and physically." Coon smiled smugly. Matt could tell the man felt he was doing a superb job.

Be polite, Matt reminded himself as he told Coon that everything was fine, and that he had resumed his work with the students quite well.

Alan Coon nodded, a bit impatiently. "Yes, yes. Well, the fact of the matter is that I have had a conversation with the specialist that is treating you, Dr. Anderson. It is her opinion that you should not overexert yourself physically because you are still not one hundred percent back to normal. She says that you are on daily medication to minimize the chance of future seizures."

The brief silence that ensued while Coon took a sip from his cracked coffee mug was barely enough time for Matt to gather his thoughts and respond, "I feel fine, Alan. I understand the doctor's concern, but when I was discharged from the hospital, I was told I could resume my work, and I promise you that we are seeing quite a bit of success in the preparation program." Matt felt a lump of desperation rise in his throat. But his indignation at being monitored by this ignoramus was much stronger, and he proceeded to outline the individual and group programs he had set up.

"The older kids should be able to fare very well in the county-wides this year." He knew that this was Coon's hot button, the thorn in his side over the past few years. It was probably the single biggest reason why he had recruited Matt - to get the older students up to an acceptable level of fitness. As Matt flipped this trump card onto the table, he watched the changes of expression in the principal's face: surprise, confusion, annoyance and, finally resignation.

"Well." Coon cleared his throat and thumbed through some papers on his desk. "That's fine, Matt. Keep up the good work, then."

Underneath the sickly sweet smile that Coon now wore, Matt could almost hear the machinations of the man's mind as he searched frantically for a way to win the point. Finding none, he dismissed Matt, closing the door a bit too hard behind him.

Upon leaving the office, Matt felt more than a little unsettled. Coon would never let this go so easily. Striding down the corridor, Matt vowed silently to prove to Coon and Dr. Anderson that despite the few weeks' setback, he had everything under control and, if anything, he was better than ever. He returned to the gym, where he had left an entire class to run themselves through the calisthenics program. Getting involved in the coaching of these students, he put the stressful conversation with Coon out of his mind completely.

There were only two weeks left until the winter vacation, and there was a festive mood throughout the school. Kate still reminisced every Christmas of the holidays back East, heralded by the cold wind and, if they were lucky, a few feet of snow. The warm, balmy Arizona days did little to put her in the mood, even though someone had decorated all of the tall Sohuaro cacti at Sunny Vista with little lights and silver garlands. Last year had been the first year that Kate had spent the entire vacation in Arizona, having gone to visit her parents the two previous years.

She and Jackie had cooked dinner for themselves on Christmas Day, and then watched old movies on television. They had gotten drunk on rum-spiked eggnog and visited some of their neighbors later on in the evening, where they had consumed more eggnog, along with Mexican beer, the trendy addition to every young adult's diet. Kate could barely remember staggering back to the house, with Jackie singing Christmas carols slightly off-key.

This year, Kate had been pleased when Matt invited her to his family's house for the holiday. She looked forward to meeting his other sister and his brothers, and to the tour of Tucson that Matt had promised her "as long as you drive," he had joked. Kate was glad she could do him the favor of driving him home for Christmas and joining him on the day.

She hoisted the box of Christmas decorations onto the kitchen counter to inspect its contents. Half of the decorations were handmade by students at Ramon in the whirlwind of activity that had accompanied the week before Christmas last year. The other half were "interesting" findings from various Indian stalls around the city. Kate was not sure how the ethnic ornaments would complement the small pine tree that she had bought, along with Matt and Sam, at the nursery, but she was glad they had decided to decorate the tree, to keep the holiday mood going even after they returned from their respective family gatherings.

The cookies still need to be done, Kate reminded herself with a look of anguish at the clock. She hurriedly telephoned Mary Sinclair to confirm their plans for baking later that day. *This is too much rushing around*, Kate chided herself, more and more aware these days of her tendency to scatter energy toward her projects like a sprinkler's spraying of the shrubs and lawn: only a little bit reached its target the first time. Her meditation was improving gradually, partly due to Matt's gentle coaching during the "lessons" they still had once or twice a week, and partly because of the process of letting go that Kate had begun three years earlier, judging the present to be more relevant and promising than her shattered, disappointing past.

She lifted the bulky box and carried it to Matt's house, where the tree would reside for the duration of the holidays. "That's one way to ensure I'll see you guys," he had remarked with a wink. Matt opened the front door, looking slightly dishevelled and groggy.

"Just waking up?" Kate exclaimed, incredulous.

"Actually, yes," he replied, taking the box from her and placing it near the tree on the living room floor. When he turned around again, Kate noted the pillow creases on his cheek, and she suppressed a laugh. Then she saw the small lump on the right side of his forehead, the blue cast threatening to darken at any moment.

"What in the world..." she began, but Matt interrupted her with a wave of his hand.

He motioned for her to sit down on the couch, and asked her if she could keep what he was about to tell her completely confidential. There was an ominous tone to his voice that chilled Kate and made her fear for Matt and his dark secret.

"I had a seizure yesterday afternoon," Matt stated without preamble. He rushed on, before Kate could make any comment, "I know I've been acting like everything's fine and dandy, but it's actually very difficult. I've had a couple of small seizures in the past few weeks."

Observing Kate's stricken look, he proceeded to tell her about the constant fear of having a convulsion, the frustration of not knowing what set them off, and the anger toward whatever or whoever had decided he should suffer this fate. As he spoke, his eyes searched hers for the empathetic kindness that would allow him to continue the story.

"And when I have one," he concluded, rather forlorn, Kate thought, "it just wipes me out for the rest of the day. I must have slept straight through from seven last night until just a few minutes ago."

Yellowstone, Matt's golden retriever, padded up to him and put his nose on Matt's lap. There was a wide, open feeling of vulnerability, as if the truth had split a yawning chasm in the center of their peaceful existence. Kate tried desperately to think of some comforting words, but found that she could not even think clearly. She resorted instead to her more natural mode, that of questioner.

But to her, and his, mounting frustration, they found that

most of the questions remained unanswered. Matt had asked many of the same things of Dr. Anderson, who had told him that the current body of knowledge on epilepsy, which Matt apparently had developed, was basically a conglomeration of hypotheses and estimations, with no real conclusive ideas about causes or prevention of seizures. The medication that the doctors had so vehemently pressed upon him involved trial and error as to the "correct dosage", the dosage that would control Matt's condition and prevent future seizures.

Kate sighed, anxious and beleaguered by the enormity of the situation. In an effort to get closer to Matt, she reached out and patted Yellowstone's head. She could feel the rise and fall of the dog's steady breath underneath her palm, and it made her feel strangely reassured.

"What are you going to do?" she asked finally, voicing the doubt and insecurity that each of them felt. "I mean, you know how Cooney feels about the whole thing."

Matt slammed his hand down on the floor, startling Kate and Yellowstone. "That's exactly why I don't want him to find out." He began to pick fuzz out of the carpet, making it into a fluffy pile. He shrugged and looked at Kate with a little-boy pout.

She tousled his hair. Some semblance of resignation, gained ironically from the meditation practice, cautioned her not to fight against the situation, but to work with it in some way. But, how? She quickly reached into her purse and retrieved a cover stick, which she dabbed on Matt's bruise. At least they could keep Sam from worrying.

Matt's mumblings about wearing 'make-up' were interrupted when the doorbell rang, and Sam's presence quickly pervaded the room like a blast of fresh air. The three friends spread out Christmas decorations on the floor, happily choosing the most suitable ornaments for the small tree. Sam appeared to gain the most enjoyment from the activity, and when Kate teased him about behaving like an excited child, he explained that they had never celebrated Christmas in his family, and that it was only the past couple of years that he had been privy to the joys reserved for this holiday season.

With a shove to his shoulder, Matt accused Sam of using this "miserable excuse" to monopolize on the fun. The two wrestled across the floor, with Yellowstone nipping at arms and legs indiscriminately and barking gleefully.

Kate watched this scene with a mixture of curiosity and relief. *He's fine, you see*, she chided herself for her earlier feelings of fear and protectiveness for Matt. She noticed how quickly she was willing to put the concern out of her mind and didn't understand the way she and Matt had both let the subject of the seizures drop, on more than one occasion, instead of pursuing it closely, with the analytical methods they both loved so dearly. Problem solving had been a skill both had learned in college and still demonstrated with flair when it came to less personal issues such as bilingual education. Normally, Kate would have loved to dissect the issue, call Dr. Anderson and her colleagues into question, find the "answer" to the mystery of Matt's condition. But this complacency, this dumb acceptance of a clearly unacceptable situation...she could not fathom why they tended to ignore it.

Picking up one of the Indian ornaments, Sam complimented Kate on her choice. He explained that it was the Hopi friendship god and that the tree that it graced would be a source of deep understanding and love among friends. After fingering the ornament lovingly, Sam handed the small figure to Matt, who placed it on one of the upper boughs.

Kate knew Sam was missing George, and she could

sympathize, having felt Jackie's absence especially strongly this Christmas. She was only mildly amused when Matt sensed her thoughts and asked Sam if he had heard from the couple. Her own sense of others' thoughts and feelings had blossomed with the awareness developed in her meditation, and she could sometimes see a glimpse of what Matt had spoken of so many months ago in the kayaks.

"As it turns out," Sam said with a grin, "I just spoke to George earlier today. His job is going really well and Jackie found work in a hospital in Denver. Those devils are planning a romantic Christmas in their new mountain home. Apparently, they've already got three feet of snow on the ground."

"Snow," Kate whispered dreamily. She hadn't thought she missed the New York winters very much, but a nice snowfall could certainly be beautiful…

"I'm going to visit them in March for some spring skiing. It should be great." Sam's eyes sparkled with excitement. "I've never been skiing."

"Oh, I have," Kate was quick to add. "It's so amazing. But I've never skied in Colorado. I hear that's heaven on earth."

"So, why don't you come along? In fact, why don't you both come? It would be like old times."

There was just a split-second pause before Matt replied. "I don't think I'll go. But you should, Kate. Everything you've heard about Colorado is true. We used to go skiing there almost every winter while I was in high school."

Sam shoved Matt playfully. "You'll come. You wouldn't miss this one, I know."

"We'll see," Matt said. He looked wistfully at a card from one of his friends in Japan.

In that instant, it all became clear to Kate: Matt must be

worried about getting on a plane because of the seizures. Or was it the skiing he was worried about, since a seizure on the slopes could be fatal. *Oh, God, how could we be so stupid*, she chided herself. She couldn't imagine a way of broaching the subject without causing Matt intense embarrassment.

The empathy she felt for Matt hurled her into another reality. Matt's reality was one of constant caution now, tinged with a little fear. Those things which they all took for granted, like going for a drive or flying to Colorado, were areas for worry now. Kate began to see how Matt's whole life had changed since the accident and it engendered in her a newfound admiration for her friend. It couldn't be easy, acting like everything was normal when, in fact, it was not normal at all.

"Quit daydreaming and get to work," Matt laughed, diving into the box to find some more decorations. Kate obeyed his command and emptied the entire box onto the floor to make sure they were not missing any of the best ornaments.

Lunching on sandwiches an hour later, they surveyed their handiwork: tinsel garlands stretched the entire circumference of the living room and kitchen, extra strings of lights swayed from one corner of the room to the other, and the tree, all three feet of it, was bedecked in glitter, and as many of the ornaments as they had been able to cram onto her sagging boughs. They reprimanded Yellowstone several times for chewing on the tinsel near the bottom of the tree, and although he backed off with mournful eyes, Matt said the dog would tear into it the minute they left the room. Yes, all in all, the scene was perfect, Kate reflected. Their own special celebration would take place on Christmas Eve, since she and Matt were going to Tucson early Christmas morning, and Sam was going to visit his family.

A light drizzle accompanied Kate back to her apartment

an hour later as she went to meet Mary for the baking of Christmas cookies. Mary arrived right on time, shaking her umbrella outside the door before entering the immaculate room. Watching her, Kate felt another momentary pang of nostalgia for a white Christmas. Oh, well, she told herself, it may not even snow back East this year.

Every kind of cookie had been suggested, some of them rejected, when they had planned for the Christmas party. Now, the kitchen counter was cluttered with flour, different types of sugars, nuts, dried fruits, and an assortment of baking trays and cookie cutters, as the two women began this seasonal ritual.

Mary spoke first, "You know, this cookie baking is so therapeutic. No matter what is on my mind, I can usually forget about it by throwing myself into the mixing and decorating." She glanced at Kate, who was measuring chopped walnuts into a bowl.

"Yes," Kate replied, "it seems so innocent, this blending of natural ingredients. It is so rewarding when you see the results." She felt grateful to Mary for being willing to talk this afternoon. "I would much rather contemplate the exact measurements of these oatmeal cookies than my other, more pressing worries."

Although she had not stopped mixing, Mary silently took in what Kate said with a nod of her greying head, a nod which was more a sign of encouragement than denial. She was clearly giving Kate an opening to discuss what was bothering her, but since the two women had never been close in this way, there was no established pattern to their conversation: they were both shakily treading this new ground.

Determined to get it off her chest, Kate blurted out, "I'm extremely worried about Matt." It was so easy to continue.

She told Mary about the seizures and how they were draining Matt's energy and depressing him. *Steady*, Kate warned herself, noting Mary's sudden frown. *I'm not portraying this properly*, she berated herself.

Holding up a wooden spoon like a weapon, Mary spoke sharply, "Don't you think he came back to work a bit soon after the accident? I mean, maybe he hasn't finished recuperating yet and he's putting himself under all kinds of pressure with the gym programs."

"The doctors thought it was okay for him to return to work," Kate spoke calmly, trying to smooth over the ripples of tenseness between them. She hoped Mary was not going to launch into a diatribe against Matt the way Alan Coon had, without knowing half of the facts. Calm, calm.

"What if he had a seizure at Ramon? In front of the kids?" Mary's words landed like ice pellets onto Kate's startled mind. Did this woman have a heart? Did she care at all about Matt's feelings and frustrations, or was it merely fear of a scene that motivated Mary's efforts to help Matt? Kate could not believe Mary's insensitivity and told her so.

"Come on, Kate!" Mary shot back with surprising hostility. "Of course I care about him, but I think he's being extremely selfish by continuing to put the students at risk." She stood poised, hands on her hips, still gripping the wooden spoon, only now with a vengeance.

At loggerheads. Neither woman was prepared to back down, yet Kate wanted the last word. "I think we are both acting selfishly by analyzing Matt's sense of responsibility behind his back and trying to dictate his actions. I mean, how would you like it if it were you and we all sat around deciding what you should do or shouldn't do?" Her voice rose a notch in volume. She almost wished Matt would read her mind from across the courtyard and arrive to defend himself.

Despite the clutter of ingredients and unfinished bowls of cookie dough, Mary thought it best that she leave. She shrugged apologetically. "Maybe it was a half-baked idea," she quipped feebly, but Kate could not manage more than a smile as a farewell gesture.

The door closed with a harsh thud of finality. Kate sat down in one of the kitchen chairs, trembling slightly with fear. She dreaded her next confrontation with Mary; then it occurred to her that other staff members might also be against Matt, and the thought sickened her. They haven't even bothered to talk to him about it, she punched the table in anger.

It was true: ever since Matt had returned to Ramon, the other teachers had begun to treat him differently, as though he had a contagious illness and was to be avoided, or at least pitied from a distance. It was not immediately perceptible, for most spoke and acted kindly on the outside, but there was fear and anxiety lying right under the thin patina of friendliness.

How could I have missed this, Kate asked herself, sadly. She knew that she had spent more time with Matt after the accident, but it had nothing to do with pity. *For Christ's sake, half the time, I completely forget about his condition.* She attacked the cookie dough to work through these disturbing realizations. By the time the last batch was taken from the oven, releasing its sweet, spicy aroma into the room, Kate had decided to speak to Mary and implore her not to mobilize the other teachers against Matt, not to cause him any more pain than he had already endured.

Chapter 10

The days leading up to Christmas sped by: too many parties, glittered holiday cards, alcohol-enhanced hugs and slurred wishes for peace and happiness. The sun had blazed like summer on the day before Christmas, and many residents of Sunny Vista ushered in the holiday in swim trunks and sandals. Kate had put aside her misgivings and had accompanied Matt and Sam on a caroling expedition through the development; it was well-received, but Matt had insisted on stopping at each condominium to accept the offer of good cheer.

"No more," spluttered Kate, shaking her head vaguely in the direction of the fourth eggnog proffered in the past hour. "Can't sing with a milky throat, don't you know?"

"Shut up!" shouted Sam and Matt in unison, because it was the fourth time she had said it. Each time, they had drunk the thick, sweet drink happily and continued singing.

Kate watched as Matt drained about a third of the eggnog from the glass, then returned it to the tray. She was proud of him for limiting himself in this way, but doubted that he should be imbibing any alcohol at all. *Okay*, she determined mentally, *I will say something if he reaches for another drink.*

But he didn't and they were soon cavorting their way back

home to get a few hours of sleep.

The windshield wipers flicked once then stayed resolutely in place. Kate hoped the drizzle would stop before they arrived in Tucson; she wanted to see some of the sights Matt had told her about. Through the misty grey, they saw a road sign telling them they were about an hour away from Matt's house. Kate finally let her shoulders relax and stretched her fingers, first one hand, then the other. She appreciated the straight expanse of highway so different from those back East; one could almost drive without thinking about it. She supposed, in retrospect, that it could be more than a little dangerous.

There was a tiny opening where Matt had rolled down the window ("We've got to have some fresh air, Kate") and she felt the cool mist reach her face. Matt had partially reclined the passenger seat and was looking contentedly ahead.

"Do you want to tell me any more about these fits?" she approached the topic casually, ready to ease off if he didn't want to talk about it.

Matt chewed on his lip with a serious look. "Ah, Kate," he sighed. "I don't want to be an invalid." She had been right about the pride. "It's so disconcerting that just when I think I'm making progress, bang! Another seizure. Am I going to have to live like this forever?" The rhetorical question rang in the air for several moments.

Then Matt cheered up slightly. "At least I can have a drink or two without worrying about it. The way I figure it is: if I'm going to have these seizures when I'm following the doctor's orders to a tee, I might as well enjoy myself. And, you see? Nothing happened. Maybe she was wrong about the alcohol."

"It's still not a good idea." Always the pragmatist, Kate preferred to see Matt follow Dr. Anderson's instructions to the letter. She smiled congenially at Matt, hoping he wouldn't see her concern as interference.

"I've been reading up on epilepsy, Kate." Matt's voice had taken a poignant tone, and she had to remind herself that he enjoyed being melodramatic. "Supposedly," he said quietly, "every time I have a seizure, some electrical synapses in my brain are burning out, destroying themselves. That explains the burnt smell that accompanies most of the seizures."

This was new. Kate realized that Matt had never spoken to her before about the "gory details". Maybe he had been taking it lightly until now, or maybe she hadn't wanted to hear. "Burnt smell?" she prompted, afraid for Matt.

He tried to describe the sensations as best he could to someone that had never experienced them. The part that was really upsetting him, as he now shared his fears with her, was that he was losing his intelligence with each seizure. "What if I become a vegetable?" he asked slowly, but grinned as he said it, and Kate smiled as well. That could never happen to someone as remarkable as Matt. He doesn't display any of this supposed loss of intelligence now. He read her mind.

"Oh, but there are signs, Kate. I find myself reading noticeably more slowly. One weird thing is I keep transposing the letter R and the number four." He shrugged. Obviously, there was no explanation for this phenomenon.

Why did this have to happen to him, Kate fumed silently, never receiving an acceptable answer to this seemingly pointless question. What could she do to help? That was more pertinent. She certainly wasn't about to bring up the disturbing conversation with Mary now. Kate felt herself fight this new truth, in an attempt to pretend it didn't exist.

She was seething with emotion as she blurted out, "You are so talented, Matt Reynolds. Don't give me this bullshit about being an invalid and turning into a vegetable." Kate wanted to look him in the eye, but she still needed to pay attention to the rain-slicked road. Maybe she should pull off on the side of the road. No, they were almost in Tucson.

Matt touched her hand, which was gripping the steering wheel fiercely. "Why do you think it's so upsetting to me?" he asked, gently. "I would like to think that I am still, as you say, talented, but I feel the effect of each goddamn seizure as it hacks away at my brain." He choked on the last few words and looked out the window, away from Kate.

She pulled off the road swiftly. They sat watching the steam rise from the hood of the car, each wrapped in his shroud of misery, Kate feeling perhaps worse than Matt because of her inability to feel exactly what he was going through. She put her head on his shoulder and whispered, "Mr. Talented. Actually, I thought you were such an arrogant son of a bitch that first day, at the tennis championship."

He pulled her head back by tugging on her hair and kissed her on the lips. They both felt dizzy in the stuffy car, but Kate nuzzled Matt's neck and held him tightly. The rain had stopped and a tentative sun was slowly making its way through the clouds. "I love you," Matt said, kissing her ear.

"No." Kate pulled herself free. "No, you don't. Please, Matt." She still felt overpowered by a confusing jumble of emotions.

He touched her cheek, but made no effort to force her. "Let's go. My mom will be starting to worry just about now." His eyes twinkled, assuring her that they were all right again. Kate wished she could just let herself go. This was Matt, her buddy, the one with whom she had shared so many happy times, sharing so much of herself. But there was still a barrier, an impenetrable wall of resistance to these deeper feelings.

She drove the rest of the way to Tucson, feeling the imprint of Matt's fingers on her burning cheek.

They were greeted by about five children of various ages, and as many cats and dogs, all jumping on Matt and pulling him toward the house. "Come on, Kate," he shouted over the heads of the shorter siblings and cousins. "This is the welcoming committee."

Mrs. Reynolds was happy to see Kate again, and showed her to a comfortable room with adjoining bathroom, where she would be spending the night. As Mrs. Reynolds prepared some coffee, they chatted amiably about the preparations for the Christmas dinner, and Kate noticed with shock that the dining room table was set for at least thirteen or fourteen people. They must have quite a few relatives coming over, Kate thought, reminiscing about some past holiday get-togethers at the Bennett house.

Since there were still a few last-minute details to attend to, Kate offered her services and found herself chopping vegetables in the kitchen. It was a warm, cozy atmosphere, with Mrs. Reynolds standing beside her preparing extra desserts. Kate responded hesitantly to the older woman's questions about Matt's condition. Pushing her own fears to one side, she told a different story to Matt's mother, one of near-perfect recovery and few complications. How nice it would have been to open up completely, sharing her anxiety with someone who would without a doubt mirror that anxiety. But the responsibility was too heavy on her mind; she had to act as the buffer yet again, to spare this woman any more pain.

"I'm proud of you kids," said Matt's mother, affectionately. "You seem to have it all on the ball. Juggling careers, homes, social life...I assume you have time for some fun?" She looked at Kate quizzically, who responded with a chuckle. This was, in fact, the first time she had seen her life from this perspective, and it was reassuring to know that she wasn't making a complete wreck of it all. *We have it all on the ball, well, that's a new one.*

"Twenty-seven is hardly a kid," she reminded this mother of five. She tried to paint a picture of the fun they had all had before classes started, throwing in some descriptions of Sam and George's parties. They were both doubled up with laughter when Matt came into the kitchen.

"Sorry to break up the fun, but I've promised our guest a tour of Tucson. We are only here for two days, after all." He tilted his head to the side like Yellowstone did when he had been disobedient and wanted to be forgiven.

"Go on," smiled his mother, "you've been a big help, Kate. Make sure you're back by three. We'll be having dinner then."

They climbed back into Kate's car, after a short disagreement as to whether they should take Yellowstone or not. Matt was right: they did not want to spend the whole time chasing after the overactive dog. Passing the Yacqui reservation, Matt told her of the countless afternoons he had spent, walking through the sandy grounds after school.

"They're a very superstitious people," he remarked, suggesting they stop the car and walk around a little. "Don't worry, they don't mind a few people walking on the outside here." He picked up a particularly brilliant stone and turned it over in his hand. "But you're not supposed to take anything," he said as he threw the stone as far as he could.

The myths and superstitions of the various Indian tribes, that was a subject that Kate had always planned to read up on, curiosity piqued by the special ceremonies she had witnessed, along with hundreds of other tourists, back in Phoenix. As she listened to Matt's stories, she tried to imagine the days when the Indians roamed these parts, living off the land and unaware that they had crossed over the border and were in another country called the United States. They did not care about these formalities; it was all one land made by one Creator, wasn't it?

A wreath of desert flowers decorated a building close to the fence, and it made Kate laugh.

"But they don't celebrate Christmas, do they, Matt?"

"They do, actually. But their culture is such a blend of old Indian ritual with the Catholic influence of the missions that it's difficult to tell exactly what it is. It would be great if we could go into the reservation to see what they're preparing. I'm sure it's highly religious, maybe a bit superstitious. Better than the commercial Christmas most people on the outside will have anyway. It's gotten so far away from the true meaning, hasn't it? Precious little any of it has to do with religion nowadays."

There was a belligerent tone to his voice that made Kate look up from the stubby cactus she had been studying. "What in the world are you upset about?" She confronted him with a sharp look.

"I'm not upset...well, maybe a tiny bit. I just can't stand to see the commercialism of Christmas reaching all the way out here to the reservation. It's criminal, in a way. The Yacquis are a spiritual people, and I think they have preserved the spirit of Christmas much better than we Christians have. At one time, I was considering the Church as a way of life." He shook his head sadly. "The Brothers didn't think I was sufficiently supportive of the Doctrine, meaning sufficiently narrow-minded and arrogant. What people do in the name of religion."

His voice trailed off and Kate wondered which statement to answer. So, this was the history of Matt's short-lived career in the Catholic Church. No wonder he was so disillusioned.

Actually, most of the Catholics she knew ranged from lapsed in practice and indifferent to vehemently opposed to the whole system.

"How long ago was all this?"

"Thirteen years or so. I was just a kid, fourteen years old. But Brother Michael had made such an impression on me that there was nothing else I wanted to do but follow in his footsteps. You should have seen me, lighting candles and singing at the crack of dawn, while all the other kids in the neighborhood were still fast asleep, dreaming of their next mini-bike outing."

"What exactly changed your mind?"

"I told you," he snapped. Immediately apologetic. "Sorry, the sun is giving me a bit of a headache. Anyway, they decided *for* me. I was what you would call "counselled out" of the preparatory program. They had all the arguments: questionable commitment, conflicting interests, mostly political stuff, really. It was a long time before I really understood what had happened. All I knew was that the rug had been pulled out from under me: the only thing I really wanted to do was taken away."

Kate ruffled his hair affectionately. "Has it made you resent the Church, then?"

"That's the interesting part. For a long time, I was extremely resentful and antagonistic toward the whole system. But a few years ago, I started to understand that it probably was for the best. I went to the monastery to thank Brother Michael, and I found that he had died about a year earlier. *That* I felt bad about, that I hadn't made my peace with him. But I'm sure he knows how I feel." A gaze heavenward.

On the way back to Matt's house, Kate pestered him for

the details about his political differences with the Church, and found that they were the same as those of her other friends: questions of marriage, divorce, sex. Matt had just been bold enough to voice them aloud. She asked him if he had considered becoming a Buddhist while living in Japan.

"Sure, I thought about it. But, you know, Kate, the whole idea of becoming a Buddhist, or rejecting Catholicism, can be so meaningless, if you keep on behaving the same way. The last thing I would want to do is call myself something, and maintain the idea that the path I follow is the only one, to hell with all the others because they're wrong. Do you know what I mean?"

"I think so." Better to stay quiet. She knew he could and would elaborate on this fascinating viewpoint.

"What is the point of getting all agitated when it comes to religion, when the main point of it all is to be a better person, practice peace and compassion...I'm not going to put a label on what I believe. I'm constantly learning new things, anyway, and that will change the way I see the world."

She could have hugged him for making it sound so simple and explaining the religion thing in one fell swoop. *That is most definitely the answer,* she reflected. *Never mind what I am, what you are, but let's just get the job done and make the world a better place.* As they rounded the corner onto Matt's street, she saw a Jeep that looked familiar, but couldn't place it for a second. Then she saw George's red hair glowing in the sunlight.

Squealed salutations, tearful hugs. Matt's sly grin left her certain that this was no "surprise visit", as George was now claiming in his excitable voice. Jackie clung to his arm as she hurriedly tried to tell Kate everything that had happened to them on the journey.

Only eighteen hours it had taken them to drive out from

Denver. They could only stay until tomorrow, but they would make the most of their time there. And how was Sam, George wanted to know. Kate recounted the Christmas festivities back in Scottsdale, fully aware that she was romanticizing the events, not wanting her friends to worry.

Mrs. Reynolds herded everyone into the dining room, to begin the meal. The children looked clean and eager, with the exception of the youngest, who sat sullenly petting one of the dogs' heads. Kate sat next to him and tried to engage him in conversation.

After a benediction, which Matt led in his strong baritone, they enjoyed the home-cooked food which Mrs. Reynolds had prepared. The conversation remained light and cheerful, with only one reference to the accident. A meaningful smile from Matt's mother, as she said, "Thank God Matt and his friends could be here with us this Christmas."

Toby, the brother next to Kate, responded to her coaxing by singing a Christmas carol during dessert and his voice was a younger version of Matt's. Matt quickly got his guitar to pick out the melody and accompany him. Everyone was in hysterics as Matt added a dubious harmony.

The crumbs left on the pie plates attested to Kate's latest success at baking.

Nobody would know that these pies had been her salvation as she worked through the night Thursday, unable to sleep because of her worries. But all that faded quickly in this warm and lively holiday mood.

The group was halfway through Silent Night when there was a light rap on the front door, and a dark-skinned Santa leaped into the room, shouting "Merry Christmas!"

Disguised though it was, Sam's voice was recognized at once by George, who pulled off the beard and hat. They clapped each other on the back, and another chair was added to the crowded table.

"How could I pass this one up?" he beamed. "All my closest friends together on Christmas Day, and the chance to visit Tucson and Matt's wonderful family." His family celebration had ended two hours earlier, and he had sped down the freeway as soon as it was over.

After the dinner table was cleared and the dishes expertly taken care of by Kate, Jackie, and Matt's sister Sarah, there was a comfortable lull in the air. George patted his stomach and suggested they take a walk to digest the heavy holiday fare.

He grabbed Jackie's waist and pulled her close as they stepped outside into the warm dryness of the late afternoon. Kate, watching in amazement, realized that she had never seen the two together like this, as a cou- ple. Their late night talks on the telephone had made the relationship seem more real, but nothing had prepared her for the twinge of happiness mixed with envy that she was experiencing now.

"What are you waiting for, giddyap," Sam prodded, slapping Kate playfully on her behind. He gracefully swung one arm around her shoulder, and grabbed Matt with the other arm. The group wandered down the deserted winding road, happily reminiscing about the past summer at Sunny Vista.

A hare bounded across the road, startling all of them. Jackie was the first to recover and she laughed, relieved. "I suppose you would tell us," she addressed Matt, "if there were any wild animals or snakes on this road?" Her eyebrows lifted hopefully.

"The odd rattler has been known to slither along here, but never on Christmas Day." Matt's face was remarkably serious, but his burst of laughter quickly followed. "You don't have to be afraid, Jackie. You've got George, right?" He leaned over George's shoulder, making hissing sounds and running his fingers in a snakelike pattern around his face.

As if in response, a rustling sound was heard in the dry grass a few feet from the side of the road. Matt advised them to keep walking slowly, assuring them that snakes did not really like to go near people, and would only attack if provoked. Urging herself silently to continue calmly, Kate felt sorry for the snake, feared and hated by so many. No, it was not a rattlesnake, Matt was saying. They don't come out until it gets a bit cooler.

They continued down the dusty road. The houses around this end of Matt's road were slightly more Spanish in style, boasting whitewashed walls and the dull red tile roofs that made the architecture so famous. They stopped outside a particularly large villa, whose wrought-iron gate stood open. The owners had planted a cactus garden in the front, working with nature rather than against it. The giant Sohuaro in the middle stood proud, spiky needles reaching outwards in all directions.

"What a marvel," Kate breathed. "It must be over a hundred years old." She could not stop staring at the cactus, wondering what kind of history it had seen in its century of standing sentinel for this house. Or maybe it had been there even before the house was built, and the owners planned the rest of the site around it.

Sam smiled at her. "You know more about these plants than the rest of us put together," he joked. "Quick, name the rest."

"Prickly pear, cholla, yucca of course and… I'm sure that's an agave," Kate finished up quickly, staring him in the eye. "But you knew that, Sam. You're the one who lived on a reservation full of the darn things."

"Don't assume," he warned. "It's amazing how one can take

the land and its treasures for granted. There are all kinds of cactus plants on the reservation, and I think my grandfather taught me all the names when I was young, but in my eagerness to learn about the 'outside world', I forgot most of it." He stooped to look at a small plant near the gate. "Now, this one should interest you guys."

"That was very impressive back there," Matt whispered warmly into Kate's ear as they started their journey back to the house. She looked at him, surprised. It was not only the compliment that gave her a small thrill, but the admiration in his voice. It all felt very strange and wonderful. She had never considered herself to be on the same level as Matt, but this affirmation made her feel like she was part of something greater, something which she had previously deemed accessible only to him.

A vision emblazoned itself upon her mind like a flash of light: a fire burning in a hearth, two people sitting in chairs, reading and pausing every so often to glance at the other, or share a passage from the book. She was astonished that she could think of Matt in this way, placing him neatly into her fantasy of the ideal relationship. Since the divorce, she had not dared to think of any man in this context, brushing aside most of her feelings like annoying cobwebs blocking her in their filmy, clingy way.

As they approached the house, Kate felt lighter and freer, ready to take on whatever might await her in the near future. She hugged Jackie impulsively, not even attempting to get the beaming grin off her face.

Later that evening, after the rest of the family had gone to bed, the five friends stayed up talking in the large family room. There was a feeling of camaraderie, peaceful and harmonious, but tinged with a little anxiety about the brevity of the visit.

Jackie and George were going to be starting back for Denver after breakfast the next morning, since both had to be at work the following day.

"Who wants to watch a film?" Matt suggested, indicating a neat row of videotapes to choose from. Kate shrugged, not having considered ending Christmas Day with a video. Still, it would be nice to see something entertaining, and if Matt was choosing it, it was bound to be good.

"No horror films," Kate said quickly.

"No mushy stuff," was Sam's comment. He went over to the shelf where Matt was standing to supervise the selection of a suitable film.

"Anybody seen *Ran*?" Matt held up a box whose colorful picture on the cover looked familiar. None of the group had seen the film, although Kate and Sam had almost rented it several times.

"You won't be sorry," Matt said. He was already putting the videotape into the machine. "Directed by Kurosawa. One of the most brilliant film makers of our time. He's a legend in Japan, and now, luckily, we can witness his genius right here at home." He bowed and the women laughed.

Jackie looked sceptical. "I'm not sure I'm up for a Japanese film right now. It's subtitled, right?" Affirmative nod. "I don't suppose anybody would prefer 'A Christmas Carol'?" There were a few groans and Sam threw a pillow at her.

"How can you even compare the two?" he pulled a face of mock horror. "I've been wanting to see this film for ages. The cinematography will take your breath away."

Matt nodded emphatically and wedged himself between Kate and Sam on the couch. He promised them that he would explain what he could, since he knew Japanese and had seen the film about six times. They settled down to watch the epic and before long were all enraptured by the story and the visual images.

At one point, Kate looked at Jackie, whose attention was riveted to the screen. Her eyes were wide with excitement, even during the gory scenes. Of course, she was a nurse. A little blood isn't going to faze her. Kate looked away during the bloodiest parts.

"Look at that!" Matt exclaimed, jumping up and knocking some magazines off the coffee table. The concubines were wielding sharp swords and were preparing themselves to commit *seppuku*, the ritual suicide. "Isn't that beautiful?" He shook Kate's arm.

"I don't think I can watch this part, Matt. I'm too squeamish." She gazed downward, embarrassed about her cowardice. "Why are we watching this on Christmas Day?" she accused, looking everywhere but at the screen.

"You don't understand," he said breathlessly, his eyes glowing with excitement. You see, in those days, a Japanese warrior was expected to defend his honor to the death. And that means when your enemy is at your doorstep, you can still win by dying honorably. Look, look!" He pulled at her arm and she looked up reluctantly.

She saw the film bring to life the stories Matt had told at the Japanese restaurant and it was exactly as she had pictured it.

The credits finally trailed across the television screen, finding most of the group spellbound, or at least very quiet. Jackie and George kissed them all and went up to bed, followed by Sam, who opted for hugs instead of kisses. Finally Kate got up. As she was leaving the room, Matt popped the video out of the machine and put it back into its box with care.

"What do you like the most about Japan?" Kate asked suddenly.

He shook his head. "It's so hard to explain. I love the whole philosophy in the far East, I guess, not just Japan. We tend to get so bogged down in the mundane in this country, and I hear people complain about the most trivial things. As if life is supposed to be easy! People just don't appreciate what they have, I think."

Although this thought process seemed to run down a tangent, Kate thought she could grasp something of what he was saying. Just then, she saw Lynne, Matt's younger sister, standing shyly near the door.

"Hi, kiddo," Matt beamed at her. "I won't tell Mom you're up so late. What's up?"

Lynne appeared nervous and bit her lip, looking at Kate.

"It's okay. Kate's my friend." Matt sat down right where he was on the floor and patted his lap. "Come over here. I never see you any more." The young girl sat down on his lap. "Now, what's up?"

Kate marvelled at the way Matt had broken down any feelings of superiority over the child by sitting on the floor, and how gracefully and gently he was coaxing her to open up to him.

"I miss you, Matt. It's just not the same without you around. Please try and come home more often." There were tears welling up in her elevenyear- old eyes.

"Hey, now. It's not that bad. Yes, I suppose I could come home a bit more often. But what is really troubling you?" He put his hand on her trembling shoulder. This surprised Kate, who would have assumed that the child had already told them what the problem was.

As she relaxed, Lynne told Matt about how her older brothers had been bullying her this past year. She spoke with the ease and openness of a child, but a streak of seriousness ran through her descriptions and Kate wondered momentarily if she had the same deep tendencies as her older brother.

Matt suppressed a yawn and Kate realized with a shock what the time was. They had been up early that day, and it had been such a busy day.

And poor Matt seemed to feel exhausted at times like this, possibly from the medication. But he was not thinking about his own needs now as he comforted Lynne.

He promised to speak to his younger brothers in the morning. "But you have to learn to speak up sooner, Lynne, when things are bothering you. Don't be afraid of what someone is going to say." This said, he took her tiny hand in his. "Promise me, now, because I can't look after you from Scottsdale."

She promised. Matt finally got her to go upstairs after giving her a big bear hug and a tickle.

When she had left the room, there seemed to be a faint remnant of Matt's patient tone permeating the room. Kate shook her head in amazement. "You should get to bed yourself, you know. I worry about you a little."

"Worry about me? Why?" He was truly surprised.

"Never mind, Matt. Just try to take care of yourself a little bit, okay?" She decided not to tell him exactly how concerned about him she really was.

He looked at her sideways. "Okay." As she shut the door to the guest room, she thought she heard him chuckle and mutter "worry wart" under his breath.

Chapter 11

The two days in Tucson seemed like an instant, and the rest of the vacation passed too swiftly for Matt. His joy at entertaining his friends back home had been mixed with a certain stress. There was no way he was going to let on how much he feared a sudden epileptic fit, no way that he was going to let it happen. He truly believed that he could control the fits as much as the dubious medication that he was still taking every day. *Mind over matter*, he told himself fiercely, when he began to feel the slightest bit strange. *No! This is not going to happen!*

It was exhausting, he mused, faintly amused at the same time. He had not had any seizures in nearly a month. Perhaps the worst of it was over. Dr. Anderson had said that when he reached the point where he had not had any seizures for two years running, he would be able to drive again. Each relapse pushed that goal farther away, depressing him. The overall helplessness he felt was eased by his friends' good-natured approach and willingness to drive him wherever he needed to go without the merest comment. But it still pained him to think of himself as different, weaker than before, and totally at the mercy of a disease that he hadn't even known much about before the accident. The stupid accident. A hundred times he had run the incident through his mind, piecing together what he remembered and what others had told him. Could it have been avoided? What if he had thought to take a flashlight down there?

Each time he started on one of these trains of thought, he consciously stopped himself. He did not want to dwell on the incident itself, nor on the feelings of resentment he felt toward C. Ramon Junior High School or Alan Coon, who was, after all, a mere representative of the institution. No, better to move on and think about the present and the future, make the best of the situation.

He tucked a folder and notebook under one arm and went to Kate's. She had asked for his help in planning a new bilingual program for her younger students.

"Thank you, thank you, thank you!" Kate exclaimed, ushering him in the door. She looked flushed and excited. "This is going to be great."

"Whoa. I haven't done anything yet. I like the idea, but let's see what we can come up with." He liked Kate's enthusiasm about new things; it always brought his energy level up too. He offered her the notebook and folder. "These are some studies that I researched a few years ago, and the notes I made to start the program in Tucson. Hopefully they'll be of use."

Kate nodded, already flipping through the pages filled with Matt's neat handwriting. "Yes, yes," she squealed. "This is exactly what I was thinking." They settled down on the floor near the coffee table so they could spread the papers out.

It had come to her while she was jogging one morning last week, that her Spanish-speaking students were having much more trouble with the material than the others. In the past, she had blamed Alan Coon and his staunch policy about integration; now she decided to take the matter into her hands and come up with a way to help the students that wouldn't cost the school anything. Cooney didn't even have to know about it.

Bilingual education was such a thorn in Coon's side, and Kate did not completely understand the reasons. Must have been something that happened to him in the past, something to make him resent the Mexicans and thwart efforts to help them.

"Of course, I won't steal your ideas," Kate had said, worried that Matt would think her lazy or unappreciative.

"Nonsense, Kate. They're not *my* ideas. I just used the information that was available and created something that happened to work." Happened to work very well. She knew the reputation of Matt's work in Tucson, even if he wanted to be humble about it. Nevertheless, she was grateful to be able to use his plan as a starting-off point for her own bilingual scheme.

Matt leaned forward to see the notebook better and soon the two were engrossed in the work. Kate was astonished to find detailed and precise notes on every aspect of planning a bilingual class. From what she knew of Matt, she had assumed that his relaxed and carefree nature would have precluded any study of this kind.

Nonsense! You know he's capable. She scolded herself quickly, bringing to mind the laborious karate exercises that Matt had been performing diligently for years and still practiced. No, he was definitely an enigma because he couldn't be placed in any category very well.

Playing with a strand of hair, still puzzled, Kate looked up to find Matt staring intently at her.

"Come on, beautiful," he murmured. "We have work to do." His voice carried the same gentle tone that Kate had noticed months ago, when she thought she was falling in love. Now, she felt a warm, tingling sensation run through her and she had to catch her breath unexpectedly.

She touched his shoulder affectionately. "Maybe a short break would do us both some good." She searched his face for a clue to proceed, but the smile was strained and a frown was beginning to crease his smooth forehead.

"Kate." He stopped. Thought better of it, perhaps? So many almosts; Kate nearly threw herself on top of him in frustration. What was this damn game they were playing, anyway? She willed herself to calm down, breathing long breaths through her nose.

Pen down, Matt sat back in his seat. "Yes, maybe we should stop for a few minutes. I have a slight headache." He sighed loudly. It was as though a mask had been lifted suddenly from his face, and Kate noticed how fatigued her friend really looked. Why did he think he had to pretend with her? She was thankful he was letting his guard down now. She leaned over to massage the back of his neck.

"Just relax, Matt. I'll give you the Kate Bennett special treatment."

His hand flew out and swiftly pushed hers away. Grimacing, he said, "Don't. I feel really weird right now." He stalked to the bathroom and went in.

Through the door which he had left ajar, Kate could see Matt standing close to the mirror and looking fiercely at it. He appeared to be muttering to himself. She let out a long breath, wondering if she had upset him.

Coffee, she decided. That would definitely be a boost for both of them. She went into the kitchen to prepare it. A loud bang made her drop the sugar bowl.

Matt! She froze for a few seconds, fighting the inner demon of fear. But she knew she had to help him. As she approached the bathroom, she heard the reverberating with thumping sounds - Matt's body hitting every hard surface, it sounded like.

The door to the bathroom was now shut; she imagined his body weight thrown against it and cringed, for herself and for him. She struggled with the door, noticing that the thumps had receded into a shuffling sound and occasional tap.

Come on! she urged the door, desperate to help Matt. It opened enough for her to squeeze in and she rushed down to fit a towel under his head. But his eyes were closed and the only movements now were slight twitches of his hands and feet. Kate rushed to the telephone and summoned an ambulance. Then, kneeling beside Matt, she listened to his quiet breathing.

If he stops, I'll give him CPR immediately, she vowed, her body tense and ready for the next calamity. It was not necessary, however, and Kate remained perfectly still, willing Matt to regain consciousness. She berated herself for her trivial worries about the massage.

Uneasiness weighed upon her as she realized the severity of the situation. Why hadn't she seen it coming? Noticed the signs? Surely Matt had, and his muttering into the mirror had been an effort to ward off the seizure. Her dread turned to anger. Matt could have shared his fears with her. After all, he called her his best friend, didn't he? How was she supposed to help him?

A dripping sound caused Kate to look up. The tap was still running- Matt must have tried to wash his face. Leading from the sink, there was a small line of blood, where Matt's head had come into contact with the edge of the basin. Kate stifled a sob as she wiped it off with a tissue. She wanted to touch him, to reassure him, but she didn't dare. She saw more blood on the floor and thought with horror of the number of times he must have hit his head. *Poor Matt. Always thinks he has to be the martyr. The fear must always be there, just under the surface, ready to be proven at any time. How about all the seizures he has to endure alone? And all the pain.*

The endless circle of worry and frustration was making Kate panic and she hurriedly stepped out of the bathroom. She leaned against a wall, breathing heavily. The lamps outside threw an eerie glow through the small windows beside the front door, landing ghostlike onto the living room carpet. Kate slid to the floor and let the tears flow.

Finally, she forced herself to pick up the telephone. "Sam...," she couldn't manage to say any more, but her shaky voice brought him running over.

The ambulance arrived a few minutes later, and Sam helped Kate to her feet, then assisted with Matt. Matt's eyes were still closed, but his breathing was steady.

"Don't use the siren unless you absolutely have to," Kate pleaded with the paramedics. She couldn't bear for Matt's pain to be broadcast carelessly throughout the community. She waved them away, praying furiously to herself. She promised Matt, still unconscious, that she would see him at the hospital before long.

"I'm just not strong enough," she whimpered to Sam, who was picking up empty oxygen tanks and torn medical wrappers from the bathroom floor. "I know I'm being selfish, but it hit me really hard. Can you imagine: Matt convulsing all over the bathroom, and me standing out here, utterly helpless? Witnessing that kind of agony?"

Sam carried one last armful to the garbage can and returned to give Kate a hug. "Don't be so hard on yourself. You did all the right things. You called *me*."

She smiled. They should have some coffee, she thought and went into the kitchen. When she saw the broken sugar bowl on the floor, sugar scattered everywhere and crunching underfoot, it all came back. "Sam!" she cried, almost hysterical. "I could use a hand, buddy."

They cleaned up the evidence in a matter of a few minutes, and Kate felt almost guilty, sweeping it all away like that. She asked Sam if they could go to the hospital as soon as they finished their coffee.

It was like a *deja vu* experience: the antiseptic hospital smell, Dr. Anderson rushing in and out with different bottles and vials, the nurses attempting to distract Kate with their soft voices and hospital gossip.

"Sam, come here," Kate said, motioning him over to a couple of chairs. "I would like to confront Dr. Anderson about this medication business. I mean, I'm no authority, but it seems to me like whatever he was taking before was useless. It was supposed to stabilize him, right? To control the seizures?" Her voice had risen to a shriek and two nurses looked over from their station.

"Shh." Sam patted her arm. "I don't know if 'confronting her', as you put it, will do any good. I've been in pharmaceuticals for a few years, and I think Dr. Anderson is using them properly."

"How can you say that?" Kate was aghast. "It's nothing but trial and error, the doctors have said so themselves. They're just guessing, and using poor Matt as a guinea pig." She threw her arms up in exasperation.

"Kate," Sam said gently, "how many more seizures would

he have had without the medication? Epilepsy is still such a mystery to the medical profession. Believe me, these drugs are a vast improvement over the ones that were available, say, twenty years ago."

"But they don't work!" She spat the words out in a staccato that defied him to answer at all. They sat there, frustrated, until one of the nurses came over.

She had a kind but weathered face and Kate could read in it years of comforting patients and family alike. "The doctors would like to know if he has been taking his medication at the prescribed times every day." *He*, she had said, assigning the personal pronoun carelessly and, in Kate's opinion, quite thoughtlessly.

"*Matt* will have to tell you about that himself," she countered, swallowing the more antagonistic words that were rising like bile in her throat.

The nurse looked at her sympathetically, then went back to confer with the others. Kate and Sam stayed in the lounge for another hour, subdued by sadness and a sense of dread.

"What if he doesn't wake up?" Kate finally whispered the words they had both been thinking. Matt had been reading up on epilepsy and had shared with them the terrible information about people sometimes not regaining consciousness after major seizures. Sam recalled now how they had all teased Matt and accused him of overdramatizing his situation for effect. They had been laughing this off only a week ago! Sam leaned his head on his arm and cried softly.

At once, Kate found the extra strength to comfort him and pull them both out of their depression. She suggested they return home and wait for information from the hospital.

"Come on," she said, tugging at Sam's arm. Truthfully, she could not bear to see her friend cry; his broken resistance carved an open space around both of them where they lay, exposed and vulnerable against fate. She expected Sam to be the strong one, as he had many times before. But, until he was feeling stronger, she would take over.

Chapter 12

The telephone's piercing ring startled Kate out of her deep slumber. She groped in the darkness to answer it.

"Hi, babe." Matt's voice sounded groggy: he must be really drugged up.

Kate sat up instantly. "How are you feeling?"

"So so. Pretty drained actually. I woke up about an hour ago and didn't know where the hell I was. When I didn't feel Yellowstone's wet nose on my face, I guessed I wasn't at the condo. Did you feed him?" he asked anxiously.

"Don't worry," Kate reassured him. "We fed him and walked him. He's doing better than you are, it seems."

Matt laughed hoarsely. "Ow, it hurts so much when I laugh." Kate's relief was complete upon hearing that laugh. She vowed never to tell Matt how worried she and Sam had been. "Uh oh," his voice lowered suddenly. "The nurses are coming in here. Oh, Kate, they're going to stick needles into my sore ass. Help!"

She laughed and before hanging up, promised to see him as soon as her classes were over that day. Classes. Shit! She would have to talk to Alan Coon for Matt. And play it down, way down. It would only hurt Matt to let Cooney know the whole story. It was the only way, she decided as she climbed out of bed an hour earlier than usual. There was no way she could sleep now, anyway, with so much to think about.

On the drive to school, Kate rehearsed in her mind what she wanted to say to Coon, who had been sceptical about Matt's condition since the accident. She needed to protect Matt, that was certain, otherwise Cooney might launch another campaign to prevent Matt from returning to work. Kate had never liked the principal much, and observing his ignorant, bureaucratic decision-making over the past three years had only reinforced her gut feelings. But, he had power. He was respected by the Board of Education as a principal who had his school "under control", and one who maintained high standards, albeit in a rather stagnant, traditional educational environment.

Kate was amazed that he had been so enthusiastic about Matt's education programs, but she guessed that his interest in the progressive scheme was mostly for political reasons. And he hadn't been wrong, Kate thought wryly. Ramon's success had already been noticed and publicized in the local press. That bastard would be shooting himself in the foot if he let Matt go. The anger helped boost her confidence and she slammed the car into a parking space, ready to deal with Alan Coon.

Several hours later, Kate was relaxing in the faculty lounge. Eddie Price came up from behind and squeezed her shoulder. "Long time, no see."

"Oh, Eddie, I've been so busy with papers and everything. I'm also working on that bilingual curriculum that I've been meaning to do. It's coming along nicely, with Matt's help." She stopped short, not wanting to get involved in the inevitable controversial discussion that would follow.

Eddie raised his eyebrows. "I heard Matt had another seizure," he said, looking to Kate for confirmation.

She nodded, knowing that would not satisfy Eddie's

curiosity. But, at least, it gave her a moment to think. Damn! She had asked both Alan Coon and Mary Sinclair to keep quiet about the incident. One of them must have ignored her request.

"It's not serious," she said brightly. "He's conscious and should be returning to Ramon within a few days." Kate wondered if her optimism sounded convincing.

"I heard it happened at your house, too. That must have been traumatic, Kate."

Kate shrugged. She had already told the story twice, each time feeling like she was betraying Matt, talking behind his back. This time, she was determined to protect Matt's privacy. Somehow, she managed to turn the conversation around to Eddie's work; she could relax now.

When the last bell rang to signify the end of classes, Kate practically ran down the hall to leave. Eddie had said he and Mary would meet her at the hospital. She was glad they cared about Matt, but still felt extremely uncomfortable about their seeing him in this weakened state.

Mary had brought Matt an enormous arrangement of flowers and now she placed it ceremoniously on a table by the window.

"Wow!" Matt exclaimed. "Did somebody die or what?" He had a twinkle in his eye.

About two feet from the bed, Mary hesitated. She looked at Matt as though his condition was contagious, and kept her distance. Kate noticed this immediately, and when she caught Eddie's eye, she had to look away for fear of bursting out in a loud guffaw.

Mary chattered to Matt about Ramon politics and gossip; so obvious was the omission of any talk about the illness that Kate was certain it was intentional. For his part, Matt played right along with her, although he must have guessed what Mary was doing.

Sure enough. Very abruptly, he cut into whatever Mary was saying, "Guys, do I have a huge bump on my left temple because it hurts like hell. Mary, maybe you could pass me that hand mirror lying on the table."

She handed him the mirror, retreating as quickly as she could without being rude.

"Wait!" Kate cried. She smoothed Matt's blond hair, avoiding the temple area which was indeed bruised and where the hair was still slightly matted with blood. She knew he must have seen his reflection already, but could not resist the urge to protect him as much as possible.

"There," she said. "Now you can look."

Matt winked at her - complicity, appreciation, or maybe both. He appraised himself in the small mirror, challenging them to admit he looked less than gorgeous. They laughed at the faces and poses Matt assumed, and Kate found herself smiling at the way he had everyone wrapped around his finger. Even the nurses, when they came in to take Matt's temperature and give him an injection, were persuaded to rate his appearance and convince him that the bruises only enhanced his good looks.

"You know, Matt," Mary began in her sober voice, "the kids will still know that you hurt yourself."

"So what, Mary?" Kate shot back, feeling belligerent as she recalled their argument in her kitchen at Christmastime.

Matt played mediator deftly and easily: "I don't mind if they know. I wouldn't want to hide it from them. Does it make me any less of a teacher?" The question fell like a stone into a pool, the implications spreading out in ever-increasing ripples. Nobody said anything for a moment.

Then Mary spoke, her tone more acrid than before. "Well, actually, yes. You can't expect everyone to act as though you're completely okay. You're a gym teacher, for God's sake, a gym teacher with epilepsy. That in itself..."

"Shut up, Mary." Kate shot the older woman a venomous look, then glanced at Matt to see how he would react. He wore an inscrutable halfsmile on his face, but was staying silent, waiting.

"I'm only stating the truth," Mary continued calmly. "Anyone can see that he's a liability."

Kate was incredulous. She looked to Eddie for help, but he was studying his nails. "I'm sorry, Matt. I've got to go," she said quickly. "I'll see you later." She gave him a careful kiss on the cheek, then left without another look at the others.

When she returned to the hospital a few hours later, with Sam this time, Kate found Matt watching a Japanese film on television. It turned out to be a video tape that one of the nurses had procured for him, knowing how much he enjoyed those films. He snapped it off immediately, saying he could watch it after they left.

Kate did not want to upset Matt by bringing up the incident with Mary, but he seemed eager to talk about it, and even joked about it with Sam: "I would say, if I were a conceited kind of guy, that I'm more competent *with* my 'disease', as she put it, than she'll ever be with her supposed perfect health."

The two men slapped hands in triumph, and Kate laughed along with them, although she worried about the repercussions of the argument with Mary. In the three years they had known each other, Kate and Mary had never been exactly friendly; actually the likelihood that anyone would approach any kind of intimacy with the hard, intimidating woman was quite small. A few times, Mary had shown a glimmer of understanding and friendliness which penetrated deeper than the usual cynical manner. It was during these times that Kate had tried to become closer with her, hopeful that they could be allies. But almost as soon as she had let down her guard, each time it was erected again, harder than before and more irreversible.

The Christmas cookie argument still cut deeply into her sensitivity.

And now, it seemed, Mary was to be the enemy once again. More difficult to contend with, for her outward show of caring and sympathy.

"Matt," Kate said tentatively, "I think Mary could really hurt your career at Ramon." There. It was said and the earth had not trembled.

"What the heck could she possibly do?" Sam wanted to know. He had only met the teacher a few times. He mentally recalled a party at Kate's, where Mary had imbibed too many vodka tonics and told bawdy jokes all evening. Sam's expression was confused, and his pouting lips made his cheekbones stand out even more than they normally did.

Immediately, Kate regretted maligning Mary behind her back. Sam always had this effect on her: his Indian-ness confronting her blatantly, like a mirror of moral rectitude. She knew it was silly, but the solemn look worked each time. If he only knew, she laughed inwardly. Because she knew he did not see himself this way.

Obviously, Matt had no qualms about including Sam in the Ramon gossip; the open communication between them let them explore most topics gracefully, happily.

"Kate's worried that Mary Sinclair could speak to the wrong people about my inability to handle my workload. What was it she called me? A 'liability'?" He snorted. "Yes, she is in tight with the bigwigs, like Alan Coon. Give me a break."

Despite the shrug of nonchalance, Kate knew there was fear underneath, but she also knew that Matt would be determined to prove Mary wrong. She could only hope he would be successful. There was something she thought would distract him...

"Here!" she stated, thrusting a tiny bonsai tree into Matt's hands. She laughed nervously. "It's not as big as Mary's bouquet, but it made me smile."

"*Domo arigato*." Matt managed a slight bow with his upper body, sitting up in bed. "It's perfect. The smaller the better with these guys, I think. Thanks, Kate." He sighed contentedly, savoring the warm feeling for his friends. He wished for an instant that he weren't in the hospital bed again, helpless, but that's the way it was. And Kate and Sam would never take advantage of the situation or use his helplessness against him, to hurt him.

A young woman entered the room with a can of Coke, which she put down on Matt's bed table. "Hi, Matt," she said, flushing a little, and Kate recognized at once the embarrassed look of infatuation.

"Julie!" He flashed his bright smile at her. "These are my friends, Kate and Sam. Julie's brother is in the room next door and she comes to see me when he's asleep, don't you, Jules?" He winked at Julie, who looked at the floor.

"Nice to meet you." The voice still had a hint of Mexican accent.

Sam asked Julie a few questions about herself, which she answered quietly and succinctly. She did not look them in the eye, nor did she ask them any questions about themselves.

Matt spoke to this girl in a tone of voice that was soft and silky, and Kate felt annoyed for some reason at the attention he was paying to her. She was just about to force her way into the little dialogue Matt and Julie were having when she was interrupted.

"All right. Medication time." Matt's nurse whooshed into the room in a flurry of authoritative energy.

"They can stay while you drug me up, can't they?" Matt looked at the stern woman with puppy-dog eyes.

"They can stay," she said with a half-smile, "but you'll be asleep in about ten minutes and it won't be much fun for them."

"Ho, ho!" Matt chortled. "Asleep! I never sleep! I'm the amazing sleepless patient. I keep the nurses up all night with brilliant conversation until *they* fall asleep. Then I do what I want." He threw them a wild look and Kate suspected there might be some truth in what he said.

Watching Julie's shy smile out of the corner of her eye, Kate felt a twinge of...jealousy? But, how? She and Matt had developed such a cozy friendship, they could say anything to each other - and usually did. They did not want to ruin it by falling in love. So, why did she feel so strange watching him with this young woman who hardly knew him?

Matt handed the bonsai back to her and asked her to put it near the window. She placed it where he could see it without straining his neck, and he smiled. "Thanks, buddy," he purred, unaware that he had just used that flirting voice with Julie. She reeled, fighting an impulse to push Julie away and cling to Matt fervently.

Before she could resume their conversation, Matt's eyes were closing drowsily and Sam tugged at her arm. "Let's go," he nudged. "Matt, you hang in there. I know you're in capable hands." This produced the desired cackle from Matt, and the two men slapped hands.

"See you guys."

"Bye, Matt." Kate glanced back as they reached the door but Matt appeared to be asleep already. Julie was still standing at the foot of his bed.

A strange sense of satisfaction overcame Kate, knowing that Julie could not talk to him either since he was sleeping. *What the hell is getting into me,* she chastised herself. *I'm acting like a jealous wife.*

"No more caffeine," Sam said, wresting the cola bottle from Kate's grasp. "You'll be up all night and I'll be forced to deal with you. Some herbal tea, perhaps?" he suggested hopefully.

"No, thanks. I've been so bored with health foods lately. What good has it done me anyway?" Kate looked at Sam with a sidelong glance. He was fishing through some boxes in the cupboard.

Without looking at her, he said, "You and I should both be thankful for our health. My God, the diseases I have to contemplate on a daily basis." He returned with a small pot that emanated a strong bark-like aroma.

"What the hell is that?" Kate asked, wrinkling her nose suspiciously.

"Lapsang souchong. Matt got me into it. Makes me feel... well, really alive."

"Probably wards off even death with that smell." But she sipped it. "Interesting," she said, trying to imagine how Matt must have introduced the tea to Sam. But, then, Sam was used to strange food and drinks from the reservation. She had drunk coffee with his mother the one time she had visited his family, but the others had had tea not altogether different from this one.

Teacup balanced on one knee, Kate leaned back and surveyed Sam's apartment. Definitely barer than when George had lived here, but much neater. She had always known George was the messier one, and now he and Jackie were probably living in utter messy bliss.

"Maybe you could get a painting or something for that wall," she said. *Or that wall, or the other two*, she thought. "Maybe a Navajo one like your mother has in her front room. I love them, with the earthy colors-yes, that would really enhance the decor, Sam."

He stared at the wall. The frown made his dark eyes look like black pebbles. He would not say anything. It was so difficult for him to accept the merest token of his heritage without conflict, since he had rejected all of it in countless arguments with his father and grandfather. That had been the only way, to break away completely without looking back. Only, he *did* look back. Each time he visited the reservation he was forced to look, and few were the visits that did not culminate in an argument about tradition versus progress.

At twenty-five, he should be able to reason with the elders in a calm voice, at least as well as he dealt with people at work. But for some reason, their steady droning voices always pushed him over the edge, making him fly into an uncontrollable rage. It was as if he needed to assert the differences between himself and them, and the more quietly they spoke, the more insistent he became.

Sam stole a look at Kate, who was sipping her tea, oblivious to the mental anguish he was going through. A painting, she had said. He had to admit, the Navajo art was beautiful. He had learned as a small boy to mix the paints the old-fashioned way, crushing the colored blocks and blending them with animal fat to obtain a smooth paste. He sighed heavily. Such a pity to give it all up. He actually had not thought about the paints for years.

"We could go up to that market," Kate was saying. "You know, where the old women sell them by the side of the road."

Careful, he warned himself. She couldn't know what effect her simple suggestion was having on him. "Sure, let's go on Saturday. We can see my parents, if you want. They love you." Good old Kate, he thought. Look what she gets me to do. He ruffled her hair affectionately. She looked pleased with herself, so he let it drop.

Chapter 13

After the four mile run, Kate felt warm and relaxed, her muscles fluid from the exercise. She stretched her arms upward, pulling more air into her lungs. *This is what it is all about*, she smiled to herself, as she walked through the tiled arch that served as the entrance to Sunny Vista.

She rubbed the perspiration from her face and rang Matt's doorbell. He opened the door dressed in a terrycloth robe and squinted at the sudden gash of sunlight.

"My God, woman, what kind of lunatic gets up at this hour?"

"This hour," repeated Kate. "It's nearly ten o'clock. You said you might want to come with us to see Sam's family and the reservation. Remember?"

"Yeah, yeah." Matt ran a hand through his blond hair. "Come in, so I can open my eyes." He guided her into the hall and shut the door. "There. That's better. Now, what's this about Sam's family?"

She caught herself before she flew at him, exasperated. He had been complaining recently about short-term memory loss. Taking a deep breath, she said in a calm voice, "We're going to the reservation in about an hour. You're welcome to come." She thought this was a good approach.

"Oh, Kate." Matt looked forlorn. "I don't feel right. Kind of queasy, similar to the feeling I get before a seizure sometimes. But I've been feeling this way for two days and I haven't had any seizures." He looked at her and shrugged, hoping she would explain it all to him in her no-nonsense way.

But she fell silent at the mention of seizures. She hated to admit that the idea still terrified her, but it did. She vacillated between feeling like a coward for not doing more that night at her apartment and worrying about the next time she would have to deal with one of Matt's fits. The teachers that had heard the story all commended her on her bravery and quick action, but they had not seen the way she fell apart looking at the blood-smeared tiles in the bathroom, how she had been paralyzed by the sugar crunching underfoot.

Sam understood. He was the brave one who had joked with Matt about the illness while his friend was still bed-ridden, and he had been a support for Kate, too. She wished she could be as nonchalant and caring at the same time.

"What's it like?" she tried.

"Like a worm sliding all over inside my stomach, and sometimes up through my throat to my head. Sometimes the worm gets really big and throbs, other times it's pretty skinny, but it's always there somewhere."

"How big is it now?"

Matt responded by holding up his little finger. "Not too terrible, but I'm so afraid it will crawl up to my head and chew on more of my brain cells."

Normally, Kate would have laughed at the image, but it was far too scary and too terribly real at the moment. She could see that Matt was very worried, and this sent goose bumps down her arms. How could this happen to someone so bright, so talented? It just wasn't fair.

"Life isn't fair," Matt stated, a half-smile confirming that he had read her thoughts. "Don't worry. I didn't mean to frighten you. It's just really weird."

"*And* it's frightening, and that's okay, Matt Reynolds. You don't have to play hero with me. I wish you wouldn't." She said this so quietly that she was not sure he would hear, so she gave him a light hug to convey her meaning.

There was a soft yet determined rap on the front door. Kate released her hug quickly, as though they had been discovered in an illicit activity, and in two strides Matt was at the door.

The clean, tanned face of Julie acted like an elixir to Matt's melancholy. He broke into a wide grin and ushered her in, performing the introductions, although the two women remembered each other.

"I've come to take you to Sedona," Julie announced.

"Sedona. Wow." The cooler climate of the artists' colony in the north of the state would probably do him some good. Matt forced the queasy feeling to the back of his mind, determined to enjoy the day. He relished the thought of walking in the shady forests of Sedona which were such a contrast to the landscapes around Phoenix. He also wouldn't mind the two-hour drive up there beside this pretty young woman.

Kate stared at Julie, slightly offended that she hadn't waited until Kate left to make her offer. But that was ludicrous, she decided. Julie knew that she and Matt were just friends, so why should she feel uncomfortable. No, it was Kate who was feeling extremely uncomfortable, rather like a third wheel, so she excused herself, urging Matt and Julie to have a wonderful time in Sedona.

As she contemplated the wide expanse of blue-black highway in front of them, Kate kept thinking about the joyful look

Matt had worn as he looked at Julie. She tested the feeling, swished it around in her mouth, and decided it was indeed jealousy. Although she and Matt had come to some sort of mutual agreement not to ruin their friendship by becoming involved, Kate still liked the open door, a faint possibility; this possibility had receded instantly with Julie in the picture. It didn't feel right, this jealousy, rather like a raincoat a few sizes too small, constricting and uncomfortable.

Sam's steady driving slowed as they turned off the freeway toward the reservation. He flicked a look at Kate, happy to have her here today. Noting her furrowed brow, he assumed she was concerned about Matt and patted her arm. The twenty or so thwarted attempts to seduce Kate over the past three years had mellowed him, given him a perspective that he would have missed had they pursued the relationship. Now, seeing her like this, he could reach out to her as a true friend, unencumbered by more complicated feelings. They had gradually erased the possibility of romance like a wet sponge across the blackboard in Kate's classroom.

"We're almost there," Kate remarked, springing into the present. She sat up straighter in her seat. "Where are the old ladies again?"

"Hang on," Sam laughed. "We'll have plenty of time to look for paintings this afternoon. But I promised my mom we would have lunch with them at one." Lunch with Sam's family was a special event, if simply for the number of people who would be present. The last time Kate had visited, most of the immediate family had been there: brothers, sisters, aunts, uncles, and cousins galore. Not to mention the older generation of grandparents and great uncles and aunts. There had been thirty-three all together, with long tables set up throughout the house (most of these brought by the relatives who also lived on the reservation). Sam did not know how many people would be there today, but he figured it would be fun for Kate.

Remembering her last visit and how she had been in the spotlight with Sam's parents, Kate felt nervous about this next encounter. "Are you sure they like me?" she asked, sounding more like a little girl than the twentyseven year old woman she was. Even her wide eyes exposed her faltering confidence to Sam.

"Come on, Kate," he chided her. "They loved you. Besides, you don't need to impress anyone in *my* down-to-earth family." Not true. But it was not important what any of the stuffy elders thought. They would never see his point of view, and he would probably never see theirs.

But the distressing part was Kate's reversion back to the doubtful, almost timid, character of a few years ago. When she had opened her heart to him that first summer, he had felt honored and hopeful. He had tried to let the bitter statements about men and the scathing generalizations float off him, acting as a buoy for her to cling to, sometimes submerged when it was too heavy, but always bobbing to the surface eventually, ready to support her again.

In those days, Kate had brandished the fresh wounds of her experiences back East, pulling them up around her to remind people what she had been through. He had not blamed her for that, not once. Always trying he help her to progress, Sam had been the surrogate therapist, injecting small comments into their conversation, suggestions to deal with her hurt. He had surprised himself, never having thought of himself as the sympathetic type, but Kate had appreciated his patience (and told him so often enough to embarrass him). Most importantly, she had blossomed before his eyes, gaining confidence and becoming, Sam guessed, more like she must have been before her troubles with Mitch.

"Oh, stop!" Kate cried suddenly as a jackrabbit bounded across the road. She smiled as it reached the other side in safety. Kate opened her car door and jumped out, ignoring Sam's confused questions. She stopped beside a flowering cactus plant and looked about to pick some of the orange blossoms. But she returned to the car empty-handed.

"What in the world?..."

She shook her head slowly. "I was going to pick those for your mother, but I suddenly thought, 'Why should I take them off the plant, where they look so beautiful, just because I want them?' They would surely die before the day is over, and that's just plain selfish."

Sam regarded her warily. "Is this the Kate Bennett I know? One year ago, you would have filled the car with those flowers."

"I know," she said. "Maybe I've changed."

Matt's influence, Sam thought, but would not say anything aloud. He was dying to know if Kate and Matt were involved, but that was the one subject he had promised himself never to bring up. It would be cute, he decided: his two best friends in love. Maybe she would volunteer some information if he was patient...

Sue Littlefoot stood four feet, eleven inches tall, but her steady gaze made Kate feel like they were the same height. She shook Kate's hand warmly but firmly, as if there were nothing else in the world at that moment other than that singular human contact. *That's a very Zen thought*, Kate noticed with interest, never having considered any comparison between the cultures before. Not that she knew that much about either culture; she just tried to read up on things that interested her.

Now, *Matt* would have appreciated the comparison, since he had majored in anthropology along with education at college. What a shame he couldn't make it. Sam was already explaining to his mother.

Mrs. Littlefoot was sturdy and capable, which was a marvel after her five children and endless work in the house and on the reservation. She exuded a positive yet thoughtful calm that Kate had admired instantly when they had first met.

Her older sister, Teresa, was even more amazing: she had borne fourteen children, twelve of whom were still alive, yet she looked just slightly older than Kate. Teresa also shook Kate's hand, helping her to relax.

"Kate!" The voice preceded the owner by only two seconds as Sam's sister Helen ran across the room to hug her. They were close in age and had gotten along extremely well the last time Kate had visited. Seeing Helen now reminded her that she had not kept in touch since then, almost a year ago, now - even though they had exchanged telephone numbers. Oh, well, Helen had not called her, either. No matter now; it was good to see her again.

The two women pushed their way across the room, stopping every few feet to greet more relatives, and finally found two chairs where they could sit down and catch up.

"How's Ramon?" Helen wanted to know, since she was a teacher also, but at the reservation school.

"Same old bullshit. But it has its moments. Actually, this is turning out to be a very interesting year. There's a new teacher named Matt Reynolds who has everyone all excited about athletics, for the first time in a long time. He almost came with us, but he had other plans."

"Matt Reynolds?" Helen looked at her quizzically. "He

wouldn't be from Tucson, would he?"

"Yes, he is. Do you know him?"

Helen laughed. "We went out together at school. Nothing serious, mostly some good talks and a few all-nighters. Study sessions," she added quickly. "Brilliant guy."

"He's very talented." Kate wondered briefly if they were going to spend the whole time talking about Matt. He was starting to dominate her life, which made her somewhat resentful. But it had been she who had first mentioned Matt's name. She thought back to that first meeting, at the tennis championship, where awe had mingled with disdain like oil and water refusing to blend properly, but rather swirling sickeningly around in the glass. The disdain had completely vanished, of course, and now she was too curious about Matt as a lover.

"And who would have thought we'd be in the same town, practically," Helen was saying. "You'll definitely have to give me his number." Her face was lit up with a broad smile that Kate interpreted as adoration, but of a different kind than she had seen on Julie's naive face. It was as if Helen's friendship with Matt, as well as their (intimate?) relationship gave her the right to feel that way. Kate felt more of a kinship with Helen instantly, simply because they had both fallen in love with Matt.

Slightly intoxicated by the atmosphere, Kate let herself be entertained by Helen's stories of her classes. She relaxed, knowing that she was not expected to say anything or do anything. She looked across the room once and saw Sam sitting at a small table with six other men; he was engrossed in a serious discussion about something and did not see her.

An hour into the meal, the front door burst open and two elderly Indian men entered the room, accompanied by Sam's father and a teenage boy. Three young children were pushed off their chairs to make room for the adults, and Mrs. Littlefoot brought over steaming mugs of some unknown brew for them to drink. Sam crossed the room to where Kate and Helen were sitting and sat down on the edge of Kate's chair.

"They just got back from a sand painting. They must be exhausted; it started late last night." Sam stared at the men sympathetically.

"What is it, exactly? I mean, I've heard of it, but I'm not sure what it's all about?"

Helen and Sam both started to reply at once, then laughed. Running his fingers through his jet-black hair, Sam explained, "It's a ritual whereby a sick person is placed on or near a pile of sand in which the elders draw certain designs and symbols. Then they say certain words to appeal to the spirits who are supposed to come down and snatch the illness away from the person. Only a few elders on this reservation know the exact designs and the secret words. They're called upon every time to perform the ritual."

Helen nodded enthusiastically. "Our father is nearly an elder and he has been involved in the sand paintings for the past five years or so." She gave him a little wave, to which he responded with a brief nod.

It was difficult for Kate to imagine Sam's father becoming an 'elder', but, then, the old men would not be around forever and there had to be people to take their place. Kate knew there was some conflict between Sam and his father and even now she could see his jaw tighten and the vein on his temple pulse in an effort to control his emotions.

"What was wrong with the patient?" Kate asked.

"High fever. Possibly pneumonia. They don't diagnose things the same way we do." Sam spoke softly, but his tone was harsh. "They don't know yet if they were successful, since the spirits may still be at work." He glared across the room. "They've done about all they can do." He shook his head.

Like a bolt of lightning, it became clear why Sam disapproved of the old, traditional ways: he was taking it as a personal affront to his chosen career and, in short, his entire lifestyle. Kate bit her lip, wondering if she should ask the other questions that were forming in her mind.

When everyone had finished eating, the women began washing the dishes while the men remained in the front room, talking. There were enough hands in the kitchen, so Kate and Helen joined Sam for a walk outside. Kate mentioned that she was going to help Sam pick out a painting for his living room.

"You!" giggled Helen. "You're going to put a Navajo painting in your ultra-modern condo? Mom and Dad will faint when they hear."

Sam shoved her, not lightly, and kicked a rock in the dirt. Kate was astonished at this display of childishness. Apparently, Sam still let his family get to him, like she used to do before she moved to Arizona.

"I'll see you guys inside," Helen mumbled and retreated toward the house. Watching her move through the hazy waves of the hot desert air, Kate felt like she was watching a film, one of those overly dramatic Italian films, perhaps.

She whirled to accuse Sam of overreacting, but saw the resigned look of sadness pulling at the corners of his mouth. She put her arm around him instead. "What's going on?"

He sighed and sat down on the small shed that held the leftover firewood from the winter. "Kate, if you knew the number of times I've tried to reason with them..." She watched his hands clench and unclench, aware that Sam's inner struggle was closer to the surface than it usually was. She yearned to repay him for the patient hours of listening that he had endured when she was at her emotional nadir.

A tiny bird landed on the ground near them and hopped boldly across the dirt. Neither one of them moved for fear of scaring the little bird. It stared Sam in the eye, then flew off, terrorized by a hawk-like screech in a nearby tree.

Such things are signs, Kate thought, her own interest in nature and living creatures greater than Sam's, despite his background. She would have likened the bird's aborted approach to his unsuccessful talks with his family, but she knew this analogy would only serve to annoy Sam further.

A different tack: "I know you try, Sam. What is it exactly that you argue about?"

"Every damn thing. How I live, my work. They think I should live on the reservation like they do, and Helen also. They think I should be here for all the tribal ceremonies, and learn the rituals to take over from my father. They live in the past, Kate!"

She nodded. "Maybe. Maybe. But there *are* some beautiful traditions that are part of the Navajo culture."

Sam's look said, Don't you lecture me, too, but he remained silent. After a moment, he sighed. "I *do* appreciate my heritage, you know. I just don't think I have to live on the reservation to prove it." He stuck out his lower lip and waited for a retort.

It seemed very simple; she did see his point. But, yet...

"You know what I was thinking, Sam?" He shook his head. "I was thinking about the sand painting and wondering if they would do it for Matt."

Sam's eyes bulged. "Are you crazy? It's a secret Navajo ritual and as far as I know, they've never done one for an outsider."

How she had even come up with such an idea was beyond him. Ludicrous. But, the more he thought about it, the more intrigued he became. It was true that the existing methods were not curing Matt's epilepsy. He wanted desperately to help his friend and maybe the answer was not of a pharmaceutical nature.

"I know it must seem like a slap in the face," Kate said. "I mean, after all the time you've spent researching and developing new drugs. But sometimes we can't see the option that's right in front of our eyes."

Sam gulped. He still had trouble with the fact that in quiet moments like this, Kate seemed to be able to read his mind. Shock soon gave way to relief and he nodded carefully. "You're right, buddy. Of course, you're right." He swatted her arm sheepishly.

They hardly noticed the sun creeping down beyond the jagged brown mountains as they discussed their plan with newfound animation. A deep chasm of hope was stretching itself in front of Sam, who, for the first time, felt the desire and the confidence to leap. He agreed to speak to his father the following day.

Chapter 14

Just when you think you know what's going on, you find out you've been looking at it through the wrong end of the tube. This was Matt's first thought when he found out, quite by accident, that the annual teachers' outing was in fact fictional because until this year it had only existed in everyone's mind. Eddie Price seemed content to talk about the event as though he had experienced many such similar affairs, his big blue eyes dancing behind the thick lenses of his glasses. "Gotta come, Matt," he urged, breathlessly. "I wouldn't miss it for the world."

"Where are we going to have it?" Matt queried.

"Oh, I don't know. Do you have any ideas?"

Matt shrugged. "Where did you have it last year?"

"What are you talking about? This is the first annual outing we've ever had."

Right, Eddie.

After too many arguments about the pros and cons of different nightclubs in Phoenix, the committee that had agreed to organize the event decided on The Factor, right near Ramon.

Matt assessed himself in the mirror for the tenth time. He shook his head, unconvinced. *I just don't feel like myself,* he concluded, miserably. He had only gone out dancing two times since the accident, both times with Kate and Sam, and neither time had they stayed very late. Tonight was bound to be a late one, or at least that's what the others were promising. Let your hair down, you know, kick up your heels a little. After all, midterms are right around the corner and then we'll have no time at all.

It was not the dancing he was worried about, or even watching the others get drunk while he remained carefully sober. No, it was a premonition, an uneasy feeling of something awful right around the corner. He leaned in close to the mirror; sometimes he could see a change in his pupils before the onset of a seizure. But there was no aura and his pupils looked quite normal. Still...

"Come on!" Kate shouted from outside, where she had driven the car around to the front of Matt's house. "We still need to pick Eddie up."

"Yeah, yeah," Matt muttered, closing the windows and giving Yellowstone an affectionate pat on the back. "You understand, don't you, buddy?" he asked the dog. He searched Yellowstone's round eyes for some sign of recognition. "No, you think I'm being a party pooper, right? I should just let go and be my old self." He gave a short laugh. "Yeah, maybe." The horn sounded loudly and Matt ran out, banging the door behind him.

Kate put the car sharply into drive almost before he had the door closed.

"Jesus, what the hell is the matter with you?" Matt demanded.

His tone must have been stronger than he intended it to be because Kate looked at him swiftly. She glared at him. "Don't you get huffy with me. You're the one that's making us late."

"So what? I don't understand what's so critical about being there exactly on time anyway. Okay, so Eddie will be wondering where we are. I'll explain, I just couldn't decide which dress to wear." The attempt at humor fell flat. "Oh, come on, Kate. I'm not going to spend the evening fighting with you." He didn't know why they were fighting; she must be under as much stress as he was tonight.

She didn't reply, but accelerated instead. Hopeless. Matt hoped she would just snap out of it. She was making him feel even less like going out tonight.

Outside the club, Kate had to park at the extreme end of the parking lot. Matt got out slowly and stood by the car for a few moments, eying the building warily. Eddie ran ahead to catch up with some of the other teachers.

"Well?" Kate stood with her hands on her hips.

Impossible. He wasn't going to talk to her when she was in a mood like this. "Never mind," he laughed it off. "Let's go while there's still a square inch or two on the dance floor."

As Kate returned from the bar with a fresh drink, she noticed Matt standing apart from the group, still looking worried and a bit dazed. The first Tom Collins had softened the brittle mood she had been wearing when they arrived, so she went over and tapped him on the shoulder. He snapped around, startled.

"Hey, relax. It's not like you to be so nervous." She waited for a reply. Matt just gave her a weak smile. "Okay, I apologize. For before, I mean. I was just concerned about picking Eddie up and meeting everybody. I guess it wasn't that important after all." Pause. "So, do you want to tell me what's on your mind?"

There was a flat railing overlooking the dance floor and Matt leaned against it. How to begin, how to begin..."Kate, you know me better than most people. You know I don't like to complain about the seizures, right?"

She cringed inwardly at the word, but nodded encouragingly for him to continue.

"I just don't feel myself these days. I want to be Mr. Life of the Party, but somehow I can't quite pull it off. Everyone expects me to be so funny and in a good mood all the time, but I can't keep up the facade. I'm so tired, Kate." He put his head down on his arm.

Kate moved to stand between Matt and the group, blocking him, sparing him any additional discomfort. She didn't know what to say, still felt bad about yelling at him in the car when she hadn't realized what he had been going through. Touching his arm, she imagined the contact would convey at least some of her feeling.

"You know," she said, after a long gap filled only with the din of the club, "I don't think anyone *expects* you to be anything. It's some idea you have of yourself, that's all. You're human, so why shouldn't you go through all the emotions we all go through? You're not Superman, you know. Sorry to break the news to you." She poked him in the ribs, which evoked a smile. "Good, so let's dance."

"No!" he almost shouted. "I...I'm sorry," he said, noting the expression of shock on her face. "I'm just afraid something might happen. You see...oh, it seems so stupid, but I've read the warnings about strobe lights setting off seizures in epileptics..."

So, that's what he was so worried about. Dear God.

"I actually spoke to the DJ about the lights. Asked him if he ever kept the strobes going for more than a minute and a half. He said no, but I'm still worried."

"Is that really dangerous then? The strobe lights blinking for more than a minute?" She grasped at the idea, trying hard to make sense out of it.

"Not always. But it's something that has been known to trigger seizures. It's not something I'd really like to find out the hard way, if you know what I mean." A wry smile.

"But, I'll be right there and if you start to feel strange, I'll help you."

He shook his head savagely. "It'll be too late, don't you see? I could never get off the dance floor in time. I could really hurt someone if I had a seizure out there."

You could really hurt yourself, Kate thought.

"But you go," he said, giving her a little push. "Look, the others are out there, making fools of yourselves. Go join them."

Kate glanced at the dance floor, where Eddie Price was spinning one of the younger female teachers around and around, with the others standing around clapping wildly. She looked back at Matt.

"Go," he said, more strongly. "I'll be fine. I might have a low alcohol beer, if you think that's all right."

"Fine with me," Kate said. "But I'd still rather have a dance with you."

He shook his head. "No. I'm serious, Kate. I don't feel right. I'm sorry to disappoint you. I'll make it up to you. I'll tell you what: we'll go out to the desert one night, where it's real quiet, no strobe lights. And we'll have a nice, slow dance under the stars." His voice lowered as he whispered into her ear, "That is, if you want to."

If I want to. God, do I want to. The image of the desert loomed in Kate's mind like a cherished photograph of an old friend. It was such a magical place for her, for them both. She knew there was nowhere else that made her feel so alive, so complete, so free. Something about the vastness drew her towards it again and again, as though she could reach out and touch it but never truly touch it at all, so immense was the desert.

I want to sleep with you in the desert tonight, with a million stars all around... The Eagles' song floated into her consciousness with all the memories attached to it. She recalled with fondness the time Matt sang these songs into the cool evening after the Sunny Vista tennis tournament. *I've got a peaceful, easy feeling*, her mind continued, the verse blocking out the loud music throbbing behind her on the dance floor. God, she could picture herself sleeping under the stars with Matt. But he had said "a dance". The warmth of his breath as he whispered this invitation lingered a moment longer.

Then a shiver started at the base of Kate's spine and tingled all the way up to her neck. Incredible, how he could still do that to her. "One dance in the desert. That's a deal," she countered and walked swiftly to the dance floor before he could detect the blush rising to her cheekbones.

When Eddie stopped dancing, the room started spinning. He walked sideways down a rounded wall, smiled at the ceiling.

"Eddie!" one of the group cried. "Stand up. You're blocking everybody's way." Thumped him with a cowboy boot. "Get up!"

"It's okay, I've got him." Matt had seen Eddie stumbling toward the bar, and had tried to make it to the dance floor before the other fell. Matt lifted the heavier man effortlessly and guided him to the door. "We're just going for a little walk," he told the bouncers at the door.

"Oh, Eddie, you idiot," Matt chuckled to his companion

who was leaning heavily against him and trying to sing the last song that had been playing inside. Hoisting Eddie up a bit further on his shoulder, Matt began to circle the parking lot again.

"No," Eddie slurred. "No more walk." He dug his heels into the paved surface like Yellowstone liked to do on the end of the leash.

They found a Camaro with a long front end where they could both sit comfortably. "Let's hope the owner doesn't come out while we're here," Matt said. "I don't need any karate practice at this hour, especially with a drunken cowboy."

Eddie laughed and almost slid off the slick surface of the car. "You know, Matt, I promised myself I would learn karate, but I never did it. It was always too scary to even get started. I know I don't look like I have the build for it, but I thought I could develop the build, you know, little by little. Agh…" he tried to wave the thought away, as if it was inconsequential, but in his drunken state, the gesture seemed more like an ostrich flapping its wings. He peered at Matt through his lenses. "You don't think I could do it, do you?"

"You could do it," Matt said. "But it all depends on your motivation. I mean, karate can be wonderful exercise and you can learn to fight, if that's important to you, but it's also about discipline."

"Discipline," Eddie repeated slowly. "Is that why you do it?"

"I practice karate to practice karate," Matt replied. "But it's extremely good for building up self-discipline, too. I'm sure you must have heard about that side of it, the mental side." He was not sure how much of this would get through to Eddie, but he respected him enough to talk to him seriously, even when the other was intoxicated.

"The mental side," Eddie repeated. "We teachers are born for that, aren't we? Everything's in the head, everything's all figured out. Terribly boring. I actually want to get away from that, you know?" He stabbed a finger in the air, then paused as if he had forgotten his place.

"That's so true." Matt helped him. "By 'mental', I don't mean that you have to think about everything because, you're right, that can be extremely boring. I guess it's just a different way of seeing things. Maybe 'heart' would be a better word than 'head'." He straightened the arm that was supporting Eddie, feeling that the other was about to fall. "Do you feel all right?"

"Yeah." Eddie closed his eyes and breathed in the cool night air. "I don't really spend time dwelling on things like this, you know. Seeing things with the heart and all that. I don't know. Maybe I'm too much of a cynic." He paused to reflect on this.

The air was still and slightly cool, a harbinger of good weather for the next day. A single lamp lit the parking lot with an eerie glow, sending a ray of hope into Eddie's heart. He leaned back onto Matt's steadying arm.

"Do you know, Matt," he said softly, "You're one of the greatest people I've ever met, Matt. I'm not just saying this because I'm drunk." He hiccoughed loudly as if to make a point. They both laughed. Then Eddie continued, "I know we don't always see eye to eye on everything, but I admire you so much. I don't know how you manage to take it all in stride the way you do. If I had to go through what you've been through..." he stopped, unable to think of a suitable ending to the sentence.

"Thanks, Eddie. You're a terrific person, too, you know. I'll never forget how you helped me after the accident."

That said, the two sat in silence, listening to the faint music from the nightclub, intermingled with the sound of the cars rushing past on Scottsdale Road. Eddie was glad Matt had been smart enough to drag him outside into the fresh air. Matt was glad he had made the effort to come out with the group.

Chapter 15

With nearly seven hundred students clamoring for his attention, Matt usually found it hard to leave the school at a reasonable hour, but this particular afternoon, he managed to extricate himself at about four o'clock. He was just locking the gym doors when Kate caught him by the arm.

"And where do you think you're going?" she teased. "Come out for a drink with us."

"Can't," he stated with a grin.

"Come on, Matt. I haven't seen you for weeks. What's up?"

He looked around dramatically and whispered, "I'm in love."

Without betraying the instant pounding of her heart, Kate congratulated him. She had seen it coming, and she really was happy for him. Well, about ninety-five percent happy and a searing five percent of jealousy. "Julie," she stated.

"It's true. She is moving in with me over the weekend." He was so ecstatic, as if saying the words had reminded him of their significance.

"Moving in with you!" Kate accused. "You hardly know her." Her primary concern was for her friend's well-being, she assured herself.

"Ah, but that's where you're wrong, Kate dear. You see, Julie and I knew each other even before we met. We're kindred spirits. It's meant to be."

She took a step towards him so that their faces almost touched. "I cannot believe you're talking this way, Matt. It just doesn't make sense. I mean, I know you wanted a roommate, but really!" She huffed, having run out of exclamations. Indeed, Matt had spoken of getting a roommate to share his apartment, after Dr. Anderson had instilled fear in him about living alone in case he had more seizures. In fact, Kate had been considering making a suggestion to him about this very subject. She knew that was the cause of the sour taste in her mouth and the half-smile she felt tugging downwards into a pout.

"I'd love you to come by for dinner on Sunday," Matt rushed on. "I do have to go now and meet Julie. But plan to come on Sunday." He waved and walked briskly down the hall.

At a loss for words, Kate followed him blindly. They met Eddie Price on the steps.

"Hey, Matt, Kate." He goggled. "What happened to your hand, Matt?"

There was a noticeable pause before Kate giggled nervously. The cast on Matt's hand was the latest battle scar, a reminder that the disease could rear its ugly head at any time. Matt, who had become alarmingly flippant about his seizures, had made some joke about rough sex on tile floors, but she had known immediately what it was. Still, Matt did not want to let many people know.

Now, despite the raging envy which had consumed her just moments earlier, her sense of honor and loyalty prevailed. "Rough sex on tile floors," she said with a wink. Eddie smiled hesitantly, but Matt burst out in his characteristic guffaw. She joined in and they became practically hysterical, holding onto each other to keep from falling down the steps.

Finally, Matt wiped his eyes and said goodbye. As he hopped into Julie's car, Kate shrugged at Eddie, as if to say, You see, there is someone. But there was a niggling feeling as she drove home, a feeling of emptiness that Kate could not resolve.

The highlight of Kate's weekend was usually a lazy Sunday morning in bed, rising only when she felt ready, and then spending a half an hour meditating. She had become so accustomed to this personal routine that she seldom thought about what a contrast this was with her previous life. Occasionally, however, she would have flashbacks to her days in New York, or even her first two years in Arizona when she used to joke, the word "relax" was not part of her vocabulary. She didn't know when she had changed; it probably wasn't a sudden event anyway, but rather a Southwest mood seeping in gradually, combined with Matt's mystical influence.

The window in her bedroom faced south, and from late morning to early evening sunlight splashed into the room in abundance. She felt lucky to have these lazy mornings where she could bask in the light and warmth coming in through the window and reflect on her feelings.

The only thing missing, Kate thought with a pang, was someone to share it with. Having grown up as an only child, she was used to being alone, and was more independent and self-reliant than most of her friends. She rarely experienced the kind of loneliness of which Jackie used to complain, but sometimes, especially in the past year, Kate felt a yawning emptiness inside, which called out for something more.

Marriage was out of the question, or so she had been telling herself for the past three years. Her experience with Mitch had been such a crushing disillusionment that she could not picture herself ever marrying again. She used to have Jackie. Kate and Jackie had always been there for each other and their friendship had intensified in Arizona, where they had helped each other adjust to a very different lifestyle. But since Jackie and George had moved to Denver, their letters and phone calls had become less frequent, dwindling to into an occasional contact that could not begin to nourish Kate's need for close companionship.

There was Sam. But Kate could not spend the kind of time with him that he would like. They had settled into a friendship with boundaries, boundaries set by their careers, differing interests, and Kate's reluctance to pursue any kind of romantic relationship. No, despite Sam's striking good looks and exciting personality, she was not attracted to him in that way. She felt as though she had given him the wrong idea early on in their friendship, when they used to flirt with each other unashamedly. Now, they studiously avoided the subject. Kate hoped Sam understood because she did not feel comfortable discussing it with him.

Kate kicked off the top sheet, which was too oppressive in the late morning sunlight. She let her thoughts rest on Matt. He was everything she looked for in a friend: warm, funny, caring, adventuresome. They had fallen into a relaxed friendship that Kate had not experienced before, even with Jackie. Because he was a man, there was no element of competition at all, and his unique viewpoints kept Kate amused and interested. They had been spending so much time together that Kate had neglected other friends and acquaintances, but she didn't care.

Since Matt had met Julie, though, he didn't have as much time for Kate anymore, and she felt hurt that he could just toss their friendship aside like a soiled towel. On one level, she could understand his apparent obsession with Julie: he threw himself into romance with as much gusto as he gave everything else in life. But it had been so long since Kate had been in a relationship like that, that she could not conjure up enough empathy to completely forgive him.

It was the practical aspect, she concluded, getting out of bed and ambling toward the shower. She enjoyed doing things with Matt; he was, in effect, her best friend and now her best friend was gone, yet again.

Kate was just finishing drying off when she heard someone knocking on the sliding door. She started toward the door, stopped, considered getting dressed first, then finally wrapped a robe around her and went to see who it was.

"Howdy, Kate!" Sam grinned, stepping into the coolness of the living room. "I am on top of the world!" he exclaimed, hugging her fiercely.

She smiled at his exuberance and pulled her robe more tightly around her, although Sam did not appear to notice.

"Well?" she prodded.

"The discussion with my father. It went so well. I should have done it a long time ago. Oh, Kate, he was so great about everything, and he thought the elders would probably agree to do a sand painting for Matt."

In her "friendship mode" once more, Kate thrilled at the idea of being able to help Matt with the Navajo ritual that had intrigued her ever since she had read about it. And the fact that Sam had broken down the barriers with his family in order to arrange the sand painting, this was truly a wonderful event.

Ushering Sam into the room, Kate made him relate every detail of the discussion, pausing intermittently to clarify the preparation that was to take place. Kate could see everything coming together harmoniously. She felt hope for the first time in months, hope that the Navajo secrets could exorcise the epilepsy from Matt's body once and for all.

"Oh, Sam," she breathed, eyes glistening with tears of emotion. "You are so wonderful, and your father too. Imagine what Matt will say when we tell him." They had not said anything to Matt since they had originally started investigating the sand painting, out of fear that he would get his hopes up and be disappointed if they couldn't work it out. But now...

"I'll tell him tonight," Sam stated. "I'm having dinner with him and his new girlfriend Julie."

"Are you going also?" Kate asked in surprise. "I didn't know it was a formal dinner."

"It's not, silly. Just the four of us, I guess. And about time too. I was starting to get really annoyed with his disappearing act." Sam had grown closer to Matt also over the past year, since George had moved away. Although he would never admit it, Kate thought he had become as devoted to, and, really, as dependent on, Matt as she had.

"It should be fantastic. Make sure you bring those articles that describe the ritual in detail. I can only explain the basics at this point." Sam looked sheepish, wishing that he had paid more attention over the past few years.

Kate gave him a light kiss on the cheek. "You're the best. Now, let me get dressed. I'll see you later at Matt's." She shut the door slowly, with a big smile on her face. Everything was going to be all right.

The Japanese food was a huge success, and Matt served up the last of the sukiyaki with a flourish. "The best this side of the China Sea."

"As modest as ever," smirked Sam, who had enjoyed his

meal immensely. Matt threw a napkin at him.

Looking at Kate for approval, Sam cleared his throat. "Matt, we want to tell you something." He paused, unsure, perhaps, of how to say it. "I have, uh, I spoke with my father recently about your seizures and we discussed the fact that maybe the elders could do a sand painting for you. That is, if you think it would be a good idea."

Matt and Julie were both looking rather blankly at him. Kate jumped in. "It's a Navajo ritual to heal different types of ailments. I brought a stack of information for you to read." She bit her lip, as Matt was still silent.

Then he burst into laughter. "You guys," he said, shaking his head. Then, more seriously, "What an idea. I don't know what to think, to tell you the truth. But, you know me, I'm always willing to try something new." His eyes twinkled with excitement.

"Excellent!" exclaimed Sam. He felt proud to represent the Navajo tribe now. His heart swelled with hope and joy as he pictured the momentous occasion that would give relief to his friend.

The three friends began to discuss the ritual animatedly, Matt giving Julie little squeezes and kisses to keep her involved. She had been quiet most of the evening, and Kate, attributing this to shyness or immaturity, was not impressed. Out of the corner of her eye, she could see Julie gazing at Matt and the sight caused a sharp pain of anguish in her stomach. *Come on, Bennett*, she chastised herself, *if you keep this up, you're going to have to excuse yourself.* Because it was becoming impossible to witness this display of infatuation.

"So," she stated, a bit too loudly, "we just need to pick a date."

"Actually," Sam hedged, "the elders decide all that. You

know, when it would be most convenient. But obviously we'll try to do it as soon as possible," he added quickly.

Matt poured hot sake for everyone except Julie, who said she didn't think she would like it. Toasting the group in Japanese, Matt downed his cup quickly.

"You're nuts!" Kate gasped. "Slightly hot going down, perhaps?" She reached out and ran her fingers down his neck for effect. Then she pulled her hand away rapidly, feeling uncomfortable acting like that with Julie there. *Oh*, she mourned, *it is never going to be the same again.*

Matt filled his cup again, avoiding Kate's eyes. Kate wanted to ask him to be careful about the alcohol, but she could not come up with the right tone of voice.

The hour was late and, as they all had to work the next day, Kate and Sam said goodbye and left. Sam did not say much on the walk home; he was obviously thinking about the upcoming sand painting. Kate walked slowly, breathing in the cool evening air and feeling just a little sorry for herself.

When she saw Matt in the faculty lounge the following week, he gave her the "dashing Reynolds smile" (Sam's words). He headed toward her but was intercepted by Alan Coon coming up on his left. In the din of the lounge, Kate could not hear what was being said, but she witnessed Matt's expression harden and his mouth form a tight line.

"The bastard!" he growled to Kate as Coon walked out of the lounge. "Bastard!" he repeated, punching the back of a chair.

"What happened?" Kate asked in a whisper.

Matt flung himself down in the chair. "Now he tells me that the school cannot be held responsible if I suffer any further seizures because I'm here at my own risk. Apparently, he's been prying information out of Dr. Anderson, and he believes I should not continue my work here at Ramon. Too dangerous, he said."

The brave expression gone, Matt collapsed into a miserable slump and held his head.

"You're not going to quit?" It was more of a demand than a question. "All your hard work..." her voice trailed off.

Matt looked at her dolefully. "I don't know if I have much of a choice. He said if I don't resign, then he will have to take the matter up with the Board."

"Oh, no. I can't believe how insensitive he's being about this." Yes, she could believe it because in the three years she had known Alan Coon, he had not shown much sensitivity to her or any other teachers she knew. He had quite a reputation as an unfeeling bureaucrat. But she had always joked about it. This time, it was no joke. "Wait there," she commanded Matt and rushed to the coffee machine.

Handing him a steaming cup-he was certain caffeine helped prevent seizures-she picked up the conversation. "You must fight this, Matt. All of the national athletics tests are coming up in the next few months. There's no one else that can get the kids ready."

She said it so matter-of-factly that he had to smile. No grey areas for Kate. Black or white; it sure seemed black to him though. He ran his hand through his hair. "I don't know if I have the energy to fight them," he sighed.

"You *have* to," she hissed. Then took a deep breath. "Come on, we'll be right there with you. You'll see, most of the faculty will be on your side."

He smiled weakly. "I'm so tired, Kate. You have no idea. I can't stand the way I feel some mornings, and seeing myself in this state...Maybe he's right. Maybe I shouldn't keep fighting it."

The confession was delivered in such an honest, pleading tone that Kate felt powerless to keep insisting. She really had had no clue what Matt had been going through lately. Since he rarely complained, she had assumed that he was feeling much better. *Idiot*, she berated herself, *you're as insensitive as Cooney*. She would have to watch more closely from now on, to pick up the unspoken messages.

When Matt was absent the following Thursday, Alan Coon told the substitute teacher to tell the students that Mr. Reynolds was taking a vacation. They did not believe his story, told with quavering voice and twitching eyebrows. They were concerned for the gym teacher they had learned to love and respect. A couple of the more vocal students refused to take part in the class unless they were told the truth.

Alan Coon, meanwhile, sat in his yellowing office inspecting his cuticles and wondering how to deal with the latest problem. Matt Reynolds had threatened to speak to the press about the unjust treatment he was receiving from the administration. He had lashed out at Coon over the telephone, warning him that the school's polished reputation built up over the years would disintegrate like a pile of sand if he spoke his mind about the accident and the unprofessional manner in which the principal had handled the whole situation.

Matt stretched out on his couch with Yellowstone, listening to jazz on the stereo. He would know the following day if he was in for an arduous ordeal or not. He felt quite pleased with himself for the way he had handled Coon. He felt guilty for lying to Julie, though. Unable to explain his predicament, he had let her believe that he just wanted a few days to rest. *Why am I hiding this from her,* he agonized. *It only adds to my nervousness and frustration.* It was just that she was so young and innocent, and it hurt her so much to see him in pain. It would not be possible to keep pretending.

He hoped she would change her mind about the sand painting on Sunday. His excitement about the event had been dampened by her flat refusal to attend; her petulant comments about "heathen rituals" had shocked and depressed him. Their first fight. Well, not a fight exactly, since they could not even talk about it in a calm tone of voice. A few days had passed and he had left the photocopies lying around, hoping she would take more of an interest. He was even thinking of having Kate talk to her.

Matt stretched his legs and hung them over the armrest of the couch. Yellowstone leaped down and started licking Matt's toes. Laughing, he gently stroked the dog's head with his feet. He remembered the time Yellowstone had licked Kate's toes, causing her to blush a deep crimson. After much teasing, Kate had finally admitted that she enjoyed it. Ah, Kate...several times they had touched on something passionate and physical, but she had always resisted. He had to admit, he still found her attractive, but their friendship was too important to ruin with the carelessness of lust.

Since he had met Julie, he had not had much time for Kate and he missed her impulsive spunk and reckless abandon. The sparks he felt at times were, he imagined, a premonition of a fierce bonfire that would consume them both should they ever give in to it. It was always out there as a possibility, if he ever felt the desire to soar higher. They would just need to be careful of the fire all around them, or, he feared, they would surely crash like Icarus falling through the sky to his death.

But where was all this coming from? Matt roused himself,

somewhat shaken, from his daydream. He had chosen Julie, after all, for her cool touch which soothed him to his core. Her soft voice was like a balm to his troubled soul, and when he was with her, he felt at peace. Opposites do attract, he had concluded, feeling like he had found the missing puzzle piece.

Only, since she had moved into his apartment, he had not meditated or done any karate kata in the mornings - he had found another pastime. It couldn't hurt, though, to stay mentally sharp. So he climbed off the couch, turned off the music and went outside. When he finished the kata, an hour later, the perspiration had soaked through his shirt as if he had poured a bucket of water over himself, and he felt alive and ready to take on anything life threw at him.

Chapter 16

The front door creaked slightly as Julie nudged it open with her hip, both arms full of bags of groceries. "I'm home," she stated, a bit tentatively.

Matt came around the corner and took one of the bags. "Thanks for doing the shopping. I would have gone with you, you know."

"Oh, never mind. It was on the way back from work. Anyway, by the time I'd have come up here to pick you up, I wouldn't have felt like getting back in the car to go out again." She sat down heavily in an armchair, watching Matt put the groceries away. "What did you do today? Anything interesting?"

He shrugged. "Played my guitar for a little bit, read the newspaper. Practised my karate for about an hour. *That* was good." He paused to try and think of a way to describe it to her, the sensation of the fluid movements coming together cleanly, the energy flowing from his body in so many tangents, in every direction, yet centering back on him again with twice the force it started with.

"Uh huh," Julie nodded at him absentmindedly, as she started to take things out for dinner.

"No, don't." Matt grasped her wrist impulsively. "Don't

prepare anything. Let's go out."

"We went out last night."

"So what? We'll go somewhere different. Mexican?" He poked her playfully in the rib.

But Julie just shook her head. She had tried to enjoy Mexican food in various restaurants but it just didn't compare with the authentic dishes she had been used to in Mexico. "Anything you want, Matt. Just no Mexican." She went into the bedroom to get ready.

In the dim light emanating from the lantern on their table, Matt saw Julie's eyes as large black pools, deep and mysterious. "Tell me what you're thinking," he said softly, touching her hand across the table.

She looked away shyly. When he didn't urge her further, she looked at him again and found him smiling gently. He waited patiently for her to open up to him. "It's that ceremony," she began nervously, her fingers twisting the napkin in her hands. "I really don't like the idea of it."

"I know. I was hoping you would change your mind and come with me, though, for my sake. It would mean a lot to me."

The waiter brought a glass of wine for her, which she nearly drained instantly. "Don't worry," she laughed quickly. "I won't have any more." Matt wasn't worried.

"Did you look at any of those articles Kate left for us?"

She shook her head slowly. "Well, I glanced at them. I still don't like the idea of the spirits. It scares me. I don't want you to go."

"Well, I'm going, Julie." Matt raised his voice slightly. Julie started then drank the rest of her wine. "I think you're being very closed-minded about all of this," Matt continued. "You don't know the first thing about it, yet you're not willing to find out more, and now you're trying to tell me not to look into it." He sighed, exasperated. "I don't think you understand my feelings about this. I've been suffering with this goddamn disease for six months now, and I'm tired of it. Here is this great opportunity to experience something from another culture, something that could cure me, and I want to try it. Hell, you don't have to believe in the spirit part of it." But, he thought to himself, you do sort of have to believe.

She shook her head. "Those spirits are actually evil demons. They can take control of you and never let you go."

Matt touched the tips of his fingers together and stared at them quietly. Should he enter into this discussion with Julie? Would she ever see things from another point of view? He remembered the strict teaching he had received at the monastery school, the immovable certainty of good versus evil that had been drilled into his head from such an early age. The times he had questioned the Brothers, he had been punished by a swift lash of the cane.

"It is not for us to question God's motives," Brother Angelo had said, with a look that had turned Matt's blood to ice. It had also been the lot of Brother Angelo to administer the punishment when they found Matt's copy of the Koran in his room. It had hurt, the beating, but only on the surface. He still couldn't understand what was so wrong about reading a book.

Now, as he cast a fleeting glance up at Julie, he wondered if she was shackled with the same strait-jacket of Catholicism, and how much work there would be for her to pull it off, layer by layer, ripping away the protective covering with agonizingly slow, painful tugs. He looked at her soft brown eyes and wished he could reach into her soul and save her from...save her from what? She had not asked to be saved. She went through life as she knew it, with insights gleaned from her own personal set of experiences. Who was he to try and change her?

He let out a long, quiet sigh, expelling every bit of air from the deepest recesses of his abdomen. He placed his right hand on the flat part of his stomach until he felt satisfied he could feel the "ki", the energy center which helped him focus his thoughts and, many times, his whole being.

"I didn't mean to scare you," Julie said, touching his cheek. She had misinterpreted his silence in this way because it was the only way she knew. As her fingers traced soft lines down his face, Matt could feel a compassion and caring that was as real as any he had ever known and it made him want to cry. He wanted Julie's love so much, but not in this way. Not with the filmy barrier between their two types of understanding. He didn't want to hurt her by pushing her away, yet he couldn't be here like this, feeling so detached from her. He felt for the "ki" again, yes, there it was, a potent source of energy for him to draw upon. Already he felt stronger.

"Rebel Reynolds!" There was only a split second between the words and the arm flying toward his left shoulder, which Matt deftly blocked with a lightning-fast movement that was pure instinct. He had felt, rather than seen the attack coming and had sent his assailant back a step.

"Quick as ever, Matt," the newcomer said now, with a clap on the back that was all good-natured.

"Not so bad yourself, Nate," Matt grinned, shaking his head. "You almost got me. Nate, I'd like you to meet my girlfriend, Julie. Julie, this is Nathan Stein. We did karate together all through college. A strong opponent is Nate. You still practicing at all?"

The other shook his head. "I actually got my black belt the year after you left, but there wasn't anybody left to practice with after that. It just wasn't much of a challenge. I've gone to a few county-wide competitions and the like. You know, like the one we went to that time?"

"God, yes. That was fantastic. Hour upon hour of the most gruelling, yet satisfying karate I have ever done in my life. I'd almost forgotten about that." They ran through a few memories, recalling fondly the times they had pushed their bodies ever further, young men revelling in the height of physical fitness.

The maitre d' tapped Nate on the arm. "Oh, sorry, Matt. I think I'd better get back to work." It was only then that Matt noticed the black apron tied over Nate's Levi's. "What are you doing here, anyway? Do you live in Scottsdale?"

Matt laughed because they had homed right in on what seemed most important, ignoring boring small talk like living arrangements. "Yeah, I live here. But I don't think we'll have time to catch up on everything tonight. I'll call you here tomorrow. How's that?"

"I'm off tomorrow. Why don't we meet here at noon? Head out to the desert maybe?" Matt nodded enthusiastically. "Great. I'd better run along now. See you tomorrow, Matt. Nice meeting you, Julie."

Already it seemed hard to get back into any serious discussion about the sand-painting. With a pang of regret, Matt decided to shelve it for a later date. He knew the misunderstanding wouldn't just go away by itself, but in the warm glow of the candlelight, in the comforting hum of the conversations all around them, he preferred to just enjoy the moment.

The taste of a carrot, the feel of a piece of bread melting away in his mouth, this was as deep as he wanted to go now.

On her side of the table, Julie smoothed imaginary creases in the tablecloth. Finally, she said, a bit wistfully, "You know everyone, don't you?"

"Oh, of course not. I do know a lot of people, but not 'everyone', surely." He could not discern any change in her expression. "Oh, come on now, Julie, let's just savor this wonderful meal and let everything else slip away."

She nodded quickly and picked at the food on her plate

How am I ever going to resolve this with her? Matt thought. He knew he was breaking his promise to let everything go and make the most of this meal, but the sadness he felt had wrapped itself completely around him now like a light cotton garment, resting without tugging, but inexorably there, everywhere. It seemed to turn into a leaden weight, impossible to shake off.

The next morning crackled through the slat blinds in the bedroom and Matt stretched like a big cat in the sunlight. Reaching across the bed for Julie, he encountered a smooth sheet instead. Before he could call her name, the bedroom door swung open and Julie brought a mug of coffee in for him. She had made it exactly the way he liked it.

"Come here," he smiled, putting the coffee down carefully beside the bed and placing a hand on her waist. He knew he could pull her down onto the bed with the slightest force in his fingertips, but he maintained a steady pressure and waited.

Julie sat down on the edge of the bed. "Not now," she smiled, pushing Matt's large hand away coyly. "You have to meet that guy at noon and it's eleven fifteen already." She sprang up lightly and went to the window. Her slight figure rocked back and forth as she looked nervously at the front lawn.

"A penny for your thoughts," he called over to her. "Or a dollar for your body." She sniffed in his direction. "We'll do something nice tonight, okay? Maybe catch a movie, if there are any you want to see." He felt bad about leaving her alone on a Saturday, one of the only days they could spend with each other. Although she had lived in the Phoenix area for three years, she didn't know many people outside her immediate family and small circle of friends. She always hung back a little, waiting for others to make the first move, whereas he would throw himself into meeting new people with the same sense of excitement he brought to most things in life. But she's different, he reminded himself.

The doorbell rang. "Hi, Kate," Matt heard Julie say. He scrambled to get dressed.

"...some of the most beautiful flowers you've ever seen in your life," Kate was saying when he emerged, barefoot and barechested, from the bedroom. Kate raised an eyebrow at him. Maybe he had left the shirt off intentionally. "Showoff. I was just saying to Julie that we should go to the Desert Botanical Gardens again. I need a fix. But it seems you have plans."

"I do, but Julie might like to go with you." He looked at Julie encouragingly.

"Mm, okay, that is if you don't mind, Kate."

"Not at all." Matt loved her at that moment for her easy answer. "Let's go after you drop Matt off at the restaurant." She was pleased with herself for not showing on her face the hesitation that had risen to the surface of her mind. It was actually a good opportunity, she now thought, to speak to Julie about the sand painting. Matt had complained that she was still reluctant to go and would she, Kate, please have a word with her? Being the noble friend was not a role that she was accustomed to. *I must be crazy*, she mused, not sure she would be able to pull it off. Still, it was quite an opportunity and she had to do it for Matt.

Seven shades of green blended into each other in the midday sun. Next to Julie was a particularly lush green cactus, appearing almost black in certain areas where the sun shone directly on it.

"I think I must have been here a dozen times over the past few years," Kate said, stepping past Julie to admire the plant more closely. "But I've never seen such a beautiful shade of green before. It looks so rich, like it's seeped in life, you know, ready to burst forth." She looked at Julie, who nodded slowly. Kate was not sure she understood. Maybe she was not in a poetic mood.

"Never mind," Kate said brightly. "Where would you like to walk, on the long path or up there where the rocks are?" She hoped Julie would choose the rocks.

"I don't know, really. You choose, Kate." Kate chose the rocks. As they climbed up on the large stone surface, they ducked underneath the rocky overhang that created a narrow alcove. Kate sat underneath the overhang and motioned for Julie to follow.

"It's great. My favorite hiding place. I suppose if people cared to look up here, they'd spot us." But the visitors to the Gardens seemed content to amble down the paved paths, following the suggested route. One middle-aged woman tugged on the arm of a young boy who was testing the sharpness of some cactus needles by touching them repeatedly.

Julie seemed nervous as she played with the tassels on her brown loafers. It would require some effort, this talk, and Kate was not exactly sure why she had agreed to help Matt, but somehow it seemed important. "Is anything wrong, Julie?"

The other bit her lip and shook her head. She seemed anxious to talk, however, so Kate fought the impulse to ask another question. The silence lay between them, possibly more uncomfortable for Julie than for Kate.

"I do worry about him so much, Kate." This came out so softly that Kate had to glance at Julie's face to make sure she had really spoken.

"What are you worried about?"

This time Julie did not hesitate. "I'm afraid of his suffering. I'm afraid he's not going to get better. Most of all, I'm afraid because I am so helpless. I can't seem to do anything to help him."

Startled at hearing this outpouring of emotion from this girl she hardly knew, Kate could only nod. She understood exactly how Julie felt; she had gone through it herself only weeks ago.

"Kate, you knew him before the accident. What was he like?"

"Well, he...he was just Matt. I don't think he was any different." What was it Julie was hoping she'd say?

Stretching out on a flat part of the rock, Julie looked up at the sky. "Sometimes I pray so hard for Matt that I feel faint. I want so much for him to get better."

Kate stifled the sarcastic comment that rose to her lips. Took a breath. "Julie," she said, finally. "Matt happens to have epilepsy, but that's only one aspect of his person. Surely you must have seen some of his finer points for you to fall in love with him." This felt really strange.

Julie bit her lip. "Of course I love him. That's why it hurts me so much to think of him in pain."

Oh, God. "Matt doesn't dwell on his condition. You know that. Why do you think that is?" Kate felt like she was being more than a little condescending towards Julie, but she didn't care. Her patience was wearing thin.

"He's stronger than I am. I am glad he doesn't talk about it all the time. I couldn't take it."

You couldn't take it! Now Kate was really getting angry. "I think you're being a tiny bit selfish about this, Julie," she said in a low voice, devoid of emotion. "If you really loved Matt, you would love him for who he is, and that is not just someone with epilepsy. Just love him." *Like I do*, she thought, bewildered by a sudden rush of feelings for her friend.

But Julie did not (could not?) reply. Kate thought of Matt's face when he had told her Julie was moving in with him. He had been so happy, like a child with a new toy. He desperately wanted this to work out, he was sure that this was "the real thing". Kate didn't know why she begrudged him his happiness. Jealousy was not a feeling she liked to entertain; she considered it immature and inappropriate when aimed at a friend. And Matt was her friend, first and foremost.

This woman sitting beside her had better treat him right. I don't think she *does* love him for who he is, Kate decided angrily. She's just infatuated with him, as if he were some perfect idol, some demi-god. And she cannot stand to admit that he has any flaws. But...Kate still couldn't figure this one out, when Julie first met Matt, he was in the hospital. She knew what she was getting herself into.

A cloud passed over the rock where the two women sat, its shapeless form throwing a filter over the glaring reflections on the light-colored paths. Kate took this moment to glance at Julie, who was looking pensively into the distance. She had an illogical desire to scream at her, to demand that she be reasonable, but Julie was still looking away and didn't meet her eye.

I don't want to be here anymore, Kate thought bitterly. She worried that this experience could ruin the Desert Botanical Gardens for her. She had tried, honestly tried to help Matt by bringing Julie here and getting her to talk, but what was the use? In a way, she felt much, much worse than she had before. It was only as she got up to leave, jumping down off the rock with Julie trailing behind her, that she noticed the teenager in the wheelchair. She guessed that it was this boy with his easy smile that had captivated Julie's attention moments earlier. What story had she imagined in the picture?

They had almost reached Sunny Vista when Kate spoke. "Are you coming with us tomorrow?"

"I don't think so." Julie shook her head, but seemed unwilling to elaborate.

"You said you wanted Matt to get better. The sand painting may help him do just that. I think you should accompany him. I know it would mean the world to him." Although she had promised herself that she wouldn't lecture Julie, it was creeping into her speech anyway. She was just so frustrated with this...this immature girl.

A quiver on Julie's lips delayed her answer. "I will think about it. But I'm not sure I can manage it." She looked pleadingly at Kate as if to say, don't make me do this.

"We're home," Kate announced, cutting off the conversation abruptly. She pulled up on the hand brake so hard that the car lurched forward. *Count to ten*, she reminded herself as she got out so she wouldn't slam the car door so hard.

As she watched Julie letting herself into Matt's house, she cursed under her breath. That night, she slept more fitfully and suffered more bad dreams than she had in a long time.

Hundreds of spiders crawled slowly up the bedroom walls, which were now turning a subtle shade of pink. As the pink intensified to a deep red, a blood red, the little spiders fled away quickly in every direction, but the largest spider stopped in the middle of the wall and fiercely gripped the wall with all eight of its hairy legs. Its eyes bulged in a horrific pseudo-smile.

Through the fog, Kate tried to escape the spider's awful stare, but she was too fatigued to move. This must be a nightmare, something said inside of her, but the reality was enough to keep her in the hazy semi-dark grasp of sleep.

Julie stood off to one side, watching the spider falter and start to lose its grasp on the wall. Despite her fear, Julie remained riveted to that spot, a malicious grin distorting the features of her normally angelic face.

Save it! Kate thought she was shouting loudly enough, but the effort was like wading through a thick stream of molasses. *Oh, please save it,* Kate whispered to the girl.

"I'm not touching it," Julie spat. "Matt doesn't want me to, so I won't."

But he does, he does want you to. Kate searched frantically for Matt, to get him to talk some sense into Julie.

Meanwhile, the spider was rapidly losing its grasp. Kate began to run through the molasses like a zombie, in a futile attempt to catch the spider. She could see the wild look in its eyes as it realized it would not be able to hold on any longer.

No! Kate felt helpless as she watched the creature begin its descent through the air, legs flailing in every direction. She had no idea what terrors awaited it at the bottom, but it sickened her to imagine the body smashed on impact, legs twisted and mangled in a final statement of defeat.

No, no, no! The spider was everything now and to lose it meant she lost everything. *Matt! Where are you?* The desperation made her tremble. In a corner of the room, she finally saw Matt seated on the floor, meditating with his eyes half-closed.

I can't help you, Matt mouthed across the room. She felt weak. Why was he just sitting there? Her eyes darted back to the spider who had given up its struggle and begun plummeting to the ground.

No! One last scream managed to escape Kate's lips as she clutched at the sheets and scrambled into consciousness. Her breath came in short rasps as she sat bolt upright in bed. Through her tears, she tried to make some sense of the dreadful dream.

Chapter 17

"Open the door a bit more," said Grey Panther in a steady voice. He surveyed all four corners of the ceiling with a keen, hawk-like stare, looking for shadows. His hands moved swiftly and gracefully as he waved the sage branch upwards in a sweeping motion.

Kate sat transfixed with awe, her lips tight and breath shallow with excitement. She had been careful to focus on positive thoughts as Grey Panther led the cleansing ceremony. For the benefit of his guests, he was explaining each step of the ritual, and she felt eternally grateful.

The sage was meant to cleanse and purify the room before any other ceremony could take place, he had said. He had lit one end of the branch and let the smoke waft toward the "dark" parts of the room. He had chanted a short Navajo verse which Sam's father had translated quietly, without disturbing the distinct rhythm of the moment.

All evil and darkness must leave the healer, the patient, and all who would witness the sand-painting. Matt looked as though he had grown up with these rituals, as he sat on the floor with a bearskin around his shoulders. He looked so serious as he mouthed the Navajo words that Sam felt a surge of pride. His friend was more of an Indian than he was, he thought, amused. A pang of guilt pounced on his heart then, for the time he had wasted, not bothering to learn anything about these sacred customs of his tribe. But that would change now. He had found the courage to speak to his father, and he would find the courage to swallow the rest of his pride and begin learning the traditions.

The room was filled with a sweet-smelling smoke and the haze brought a vague sense of unreality to the proceedings. Or maybe he was fainting. Matt leaned forward and opened his eyes wider. Kate caught his eye and gave him a warm smile.

How brave he looks, she thought fondly. And brave it was, indeed, to step into a ritual such as this with no experience of it whatsoever. During the sand painting, she had read, all kinds of spirits would be hovering around Matt's body, ready to heal him or hurt him at the slightest change in mood. Well, she didn't know how much of that she believed, but it sure was convincing, sitting in the lodge with the Navajos in their traditional dress and the smell of the burning sage.

Grey Panther and another elder were now taking jars of sand and placing them in a semicircle near Matt. There was a large animal skin that lay smooth side up in the middle of the floor, ready to receive the colored sands.

Kate reached out and squeezed Sam's hand in excitement. He shook her hand away roughly then bit his lip. *Can't do that,* he mouthed, with a quick smile to apologize for his roughness.

Each participant was asked to be involved in some way in the healing ritual. Kate was handed a tall, white candle by the only other woman present, a middle-aged Navajo wearing what looked like a hundred necklaces of small carved animal shapes. Kate looked at the other woman, awaiting further instructions, but when given none, she held the candle out in front of her, where it illuminated Matt's face and upper body. The woman smiled slightly and nodded almost imperceptibly.

The next three hours produced a mood of watchful stillness, as Grey Panther invoked the good spirits to come down and drape a cloak of healing over Matt, as he was draping sand, bit by bit, over the animal skin. For a brief instant, Kate imagined that the grains sifting through his gnarled fingers were glowing, but she quickly caught herself and blamed her fanciful imagination and the slow chanting which was mesmerizing her. When she saw a shadowy form pass across Matt's face, she just stared in disbelief. Without moving her head, she lifted her eyes to look at Sam, but he was concentrating on the chanting.

The ceremony stretched out throughout the warm afternoon, winding its way around the group like a passionate embrace. When Grey Panther finally held up his empty hands to signify the end, Kate felt riveted to her seat, unable to move. She tested her breath, first a shallow one, then a long heaving one, almost like a shuddering sigh, which seemed to loosen her limbs again.

Words seemed trivial after the chanting and periods of silence. There was nothing she wanted to say to Sam so she just smiled, relishing the perfect calm of the moment. Matt had fallen asleep, presumably from sheer exhaustion. He lay curled up like a cat on the bearskin.

After forty minutes of quiet walking around the reservation, Kate and Sam stopped beside a small creek. The water ran thinly toward the fence that marked the edge of the reservation.

"It was good," Sam remarked thoughtfully. "It felt like we were all really present, all moving together to make something happen."

Kate swallowed hard and nodded. She could not yet voice

the emotion that she felt, an emotion as complex as any she had ever experienced, with elements of richness and wonder, ecstasy and fear at once. She felt as though if she spoke about it, the entire feeling would evaporate, leaving them at the mercy of some unknown fate.

The images created during the ceremony remained very vivid in Kate's mind, especially the shadows. She recalled a recent conversation with Matt where he kept describing the epilepsy as a shadow that always hovered nearby, sometimes eclipsing his body completely (during the fits) but most of the time casting a dark tint over his heart that was a constant reminder of his fragility. Kate pondered over this idea of the shadow, stretching her own arm out in front of her to see what kind of shadow the late afternoon sun would add.

"Pity Julie couldn't make it," Sam said suddenly. The statement was so abrupt and disruptive to Kate's pensive state that she whirled on her friend with a glare.

"She *wouldn't* come. Didn't he tell you? I just can't believe anyone could be so insensitive. I tried to talk to her yesterday, but she is very religious and she wouldn't feel comfortable at a ceremony like this. Never mind the fact that Matt really would have wanted her here." The meditative mood of the past few hours had been shattered and replaced by the strong anger that had begun to boil inside her the day before. There was a bitter taste in her mouth that made her want to spit.

"What in the world..." Sam looked at her quizzically, shaking his head slightly. "I don't have any idea what is going on. All I know is Matt said Julie couldn't join us." He again looked at Kate for an explanation.

"Never mind now, Sam." Kate felt a desire to nudge the mood back to where it had been. She smiled tentatively and took Sam's arm. "Come on. Let's go back and see if Superman is awake yet."

Back at Sam's house, there was a large group of people in the front room, some seated on chairs, but most half-stretched out on the floor. Matt was seated against a wall, holding a mug of tea and talking to the group. He appeared to be in the middle of a story, having captured the attention of the group.

"But the snake didn't hear me approach," he said now, pausing to let the intrigue and suspense take effect. "I got my left hand around the top of his head and quickly shoved the stick in his mouth. The way his teeth clamped down on that stick gave me the chills. Could have been my damn arm!"

At this point, some of the Indians chuckled softly at the cowboy-like expression. One of the women refilled his cup and nobody looked interested in going anywhere.

Matt saw Kate and Sam enter and waved them over happily. As they settled on the floor next to him, he put his arms around them affectionately. Helen took a step toward them, hesitated, then practically flew over. She held a small package in front of her, proffering it to Matt.

Tearing the paper carefully, Matt revealed a small stone figurine. "A bear." He smiled, holding it up for the others to see the carved figure's simple beauty.

"We call it a fetish," Helen explained shyly. "It's actually a Zuni figure. It is supposed to protect you and give you some of the bear's strength. All you need to do is take care of it."

Matt held the fetish tenderly and thanked Helen. There were nods and murmurs of approval from the Indians gathered around them. Matt moved over slightly to make room for Helen to sit down, and Kate noticed the effort with which he shifted his weight.

"Are you all right?" she whispered, alarmed.

Matt rolled his eyes. "Of course I'm all right. Just a bit tired, that's all." He shoved her playfully and she realized they would not be able to discuss it until later.

Sam's father beckoned to Sam and they left the house a few moments later. Matt placed the bear fetish on the rug where Sam had been sitting and leaned in to the group, which by now was mostly women.

After seeing Sam leave with his father and Matt make himself comfortable again, Kate relaxed and sipped the herbal tea that Mrs. Littlefoot had given her. Gradually the warmth returned and Kate let the mood take over. She felt no desire to take part in the conversation which Helen was starting about modern education, and although this surprised her, she noted vaguely that it was not apathy that caused her to retreat, but rather a sense that it was not really necessary to say anything. Some kind of peace and tranquility that she had never quite experienced before. As she listened to Helen expound vehemently about the inequalities between public schools and reservation schools, Kate savored her observations with a neat detachedness that made her smile.

An hour and a half later, the group dispersed, Kate, Matt and Sam taking their leave from the Littlefoot family and friends. Kate was glad she had let Sam drive because in her meditative state, she felt reluctant to concentrate on the road.

Matt surprised them both when he asked about halfway back to Scottsdale, "What do you guys think of Julie?"

Looking at him in the rearview mirror, Kate saw the intent stare that was so characteristic of her friend. She wondered if this was another example of his keen awareness of her thoughts. "She's nice, Matt," she offered.

"Come on, Kate. That's not the answer I'm looking for. You've made some comments over the past few weeks that make me wonder what you're thinking. We're friends, you can tell me. I really want to know." He softened the demand with a light touch on her arm that made her want to cry for some strange reason.

"Oh, Matt," she began, not knowing exactly what to say. "I'm glad you met Julie because she seems to make you happy. You have been pretty happy lately, so I know she must be doing something right." (Wicked grin from Matt). Kate debated whether or not to continue, and upon seeing Sam's glance decided to open up about her concern.

"I don't like the fact that she didn't come today. It's not right. If she loves you, she should be here."

The caustic response Kate was expecting did not come. Instead, Matt let out a heavy sigh and nodded. "I agree. I tried to get her to come, but she didn't want to. I'm not sure exactly what she's afraid of, but it has something to do with her religion."

"Her religion?" Sam piped up. "I thought she was Catholic like you are."

"She is," Matt agreed. "But the Mexican Catholics are a lot more superstitious than we are. The idea of the spirits was a bit much for her. I may be a Catholic, but I think you'd agree, I am open to different ideas," he finished defiantly.

"You are," Sam said quickly, thankful that Matt was sharing his problem with them of his own accord. "Maybe you'll be able to explain to her how it went today so she'll be able to understand a bit better."

"Maybe." Matt didn't sound convinced.

Kate turned around in her seat so she could look at Matt. "Now, don't take this the wrong way."

"Oh, God."

"No, come on. I just wanted to ask you how on earth you

decided to let her move in with you when you hardly knew each other at all? That's what gets me. There are probably so many things you don't know about each other."

Matt sighed again. "I hadn't met someone like Julie in so long. She's so sweet and pretty and we have such a good time together. You're right, Kate, there are many things we need to learn about each other, but when you're in love, you don't think about these things."

In love? In love?!!! Kate took a couple of deep breaths before she said anything. It really hurt, hearing him say those words.

"How about the fact that actions have consequences?" she asked softly. "You were the one who taught me that. Believe me, I know how you feel. At least, I think I do. It's just that Sam and I care about you and we don't want to see you get hurt." She hoped Sam didn't mind her including him in her argument.

They had reached Scottsdale and were approaching the Sunny Vista apartments. Kate wished she had more time to explain to Matt what she meant. "If you want to talk more, I'll be around most of this week. I've got all the students' research papers to correct."

"Thanks, Kate." Matt flashed his best glamor smile at her as he shook himself free of the seat belt. She found it hard to believe that just a few hours earlier, he had lain on a bearskin rug, exhausted from the rites of a Navajo healing ceremony.

"Where's the bear fetish Helen gave you?" she asked.

"Right here, don't worry." He held the figure in the palm of his hand and stroked its back lovingly. "This bundle tied to the back, that's what holds the power. This guy is definitely going to bring me some luck."

The figure seemed to glow in the mellow light cast by the streetlamps in the parking area. The three exited Sam's car quietly, sensing that the day was indeed over.

"Tennis on Tuesday, Matt. No excuses." Sam wagged a finger at his friend who, since becoming involved with Julie, had cancelled most of their games.

"You're on," Matt replied. He then gave each of them a lingering hug before retreating to his apartment.

After he had gone, Kate and Sam remained by the car. Kate watched a neighbor's cat stalk imaginary prey in the dim light. It filled her with a vague sense of discomfort.

"Do you think he'll be all right?" she asked, subdued by her own doubts.

Sam shrugged. "Too early to tell. He certainly seems uplifted and strong. But then, I always see Matt that way." He tousled Kate's hair. "Don't fret about it now. There's nothing left to do, except let nature take its course." He smiled. "The spirits are on his side, I'm sure." Then, more playfully: "So you liked the ceremony?"

"Liked it? I was in heaven, I think. I've never seen or heard anything more mesmerizing and beautiful." The words were still inadequate to describe the effect the sand painting had had on her.

"Good. I'm pleased. Now, let's get some sleep. It's been a long day."

Kate glanced at him quickly and he burst out laughing.

"No, you idiot. I'm not propositioning you. You go sleep in your own bed. Unless you're afraid the spirits will haunt your sleep."

She waved him away. "I'll be fine. Thanks for driving today, by the way. I wasn't up to it."

"No problem. Good night, Kate."

"Good night." As she walked toward her apartment, she stopped suddenly and called him back.

"Hey, Sam, what did your father want, anyway?"

Sam looked at the ground briefly and Kate thought she saw a blush rise to his high cheekbones. "Basically, he just thanked me for making the effort to get involved on the reservation again. He's not a man of many words, but I think he was saying he's proud of me."

She hugged him tightly. "I'm proud of you, too," she said softly in a voice that was hoarse with emotion. "I'm definitely proud of you."

Chapter 18

"I don't believe it!" Kate shrieked down the phone line. "Twins, Jackie! I'm so jealous. No, I'm not. Yes, I am. Well, you know..." her voice broke into a cascade of giggles.

Jackie and George had telephoned her three months ago from a hotel in Reno, where they had gone to get married. The big wedding was no longer important, Jackie had decided, since she had discovered she was pregnant. Kate was ecstatic for her friend, if slightly disappointed at missing a chance to witness the event. And now, the ultrasound had revealed two heartbeats, and Jackie and George were preparing two cribs in the newly finished nursery.

"I don't know what to say, Jack." Kate wished she could abandon her classes and jump on the next plane to Denver. "I am really, really happy for you. Two babies, wow. And I'm nowhere near having even one. I know, I know, plenty of time yet, but I will be thirty in a couple of years...My love life? What love life? No, I surround myself with good-looking men like Matt and Sam, so it looks like I'm desirable...No, I'm serious, there's no one."

Kate tried to explain to Jackie all of the major events of the past few months and found herself talking almost exclusively about Matt. Because the two women had been so close over the years, there was a silent understanding, a reading between the lines that characterized all of their conversations. This one was no different, and Kate had barely said anything when Jackie pounced and asked her when she and Matt were finally going to "shack up together".

"Come on, Jackie. It's not like that. We're buddies, you know that. Besides, he's just split up with someone he thought was his dream girl. No, you don't know her. They met in the hospital and the whole affair has only lasted about a month... Jackie! Call him yourself if you want the details. I am not spending this time on the phone with you talking about Matt Reynolds!"

When she finally hung up the phone a half hour later, Kate tried to go back to the papers she had been correcting, but found she couldn't concentrate. She flung the pen across the room in frustration and went outside.

Matt's door was unlocked, as usual, so after a light knock, she went in. She had scolded him a few times about being so careless, but he had reminded her that he could do with some karate practice.

"Are you there?" she asked tentatively, feeling like an intruder despite Matt's constant urging to make herself at home.

"In here," a muffled voice came from the bathroom. Seconds later, Matt emerged, looking wan. Before she could say anything, he pointed to the bathroom floor, where two large towels were trying to soak up a puddle of water.

"Focal seizure, I think. Hell, I don't know. All I know is I was filling up the basin to wash my face and the next thing I know, the water is overflowing onto the floor. Must have been going for a few minutes." He shrugged.

"Oh, God, Matt." Not again, she wanted to say. She went to touch him, but he moved aside violently to avoid her.

"Don't. I'm all right." He threw another towel onto the bathroom floor on top of the two drenched ones. "So, how are you, anyway?"

Kate was surprised and hurt by Matt's brusqueness. She understood that he did not want to be babied, but it wasn't like him to jump down her throat like that. She had to remind herself that he was under a lot of stress, not the least of which being physical. Softening, she told him about Jackie and George, and they enjoyed a good-natured laugh at their friends' expense.

The mood was light for about thirty seconds before tears welled up in Matt's eyes. "I thought Julie and I were going to be together for a long time and get married and have lots of babies." He cast a mournful look her way before continuing. "I don't know why we couldn't work it out. She was just too scared, I think. I'm a bit much for a girl like that, I guess." He choked on a half-hearted laugh.

Kate did not feel comfortable responding since she was secretly glad Matt and Julie had parted ways. She had nothing against the girl; it was just that she thought her friend should have someone better. She couldn't possibly tell Matt that she had seen this coming.

"Did you ever have a seizure in front of her?" The question was out before Kate could figure out why she was so curious about it. Maybe because then she would be able to empathize a bit more with Julie.

"Not exactly. There was the one time when I think I had a seizure in bed, a couple of weeks ago. Julie was sleeping and I was going to tell her I thought I felt one coming on, but I sort of blacked out. Maybe it was a seizure, maybe not." Matt looked pensive.

"Now I'm intrigued," Kate replied. "You can tell when

you're about to have one?" That meant that perhaps he could begin to understand what was causing them.

Matt shook his head. "Only sometimes. There's a sort of burnt smell, I think I told you about it. But, most of the time, by the time I smell that, it's too late." He went on to describe the worm-like feeling that still plagued him most of the time. From what he was telling her, the worm had become more like a large serpent over the past few months.

Afraid of the answer, Kate hesitantly asked him if he had noticed any difference since the sand painting two weeks earlier.

"I think so. Maybe it's just mind over matter, but I don't care, so long as I don't have as many seizures. I can't remember exactly what Sam's father said, can you? You know, the part about waiting to see the effects, that 'settling period'?"

According to Mr. Littlefoot, Kate said, Matt should have known by now if the healing had been successful. Seeing the disappointment envelop his face, she quickly added that the effects were probably long-lasting and that they should not assume that his present condition would continue on the same course at all.

During the next week, Kate hardly lifted her head from the seemingly bottomless pile of uncorrected research papers (why did it seem like the students' writing was getting worse each year? Or maybe she hadn't done her job properly... never mind the guilt trip, Bennett, just get on with the marking).

On a particularly discouraging afternoon when she was just about to give up, the door to her classroom burst open and Eddie Price marched in.

"Now he's really done it," Eddie said in an amazed tone. "What has gotten into him, anyway?" As he stood near Kate's desk, shaking his head, she closed her books and asked him to explain.

"Why, Matt, of course. He confronted Alan Coon about the threat to take some of his classes away. Didn't you hear?"

"I've been busy, Eddie. I've got these papers to mark. So, I haven't seen or heard from Matt in a while. What threat are you talking about?" She fought to keep her voice calm, despite the wave of fear rising inside her.

Eddie furiously picked lint off his dark shirt as he explained. "Ever since the seizure in February, Coon has been trying to nail Matt to the wall with his bureaucratic bullshit. He let up for a few weeks when Matt was considering going to the Board of Education himself to complain about unfair treatment."

"Yes, I remember," Kate nodded, recalling the incidents that had punctuated the early part of the term. "And Coon wasn't interested in calling attention to himself or the school, right?"

"Right. At least, that's how it seemed. But, apparently he has decided to take the risk because he informed Matt yesterday that they would be having a substitute teacher do seven of his ten classes starting next month." Kate eyes widened in horror. "So, what does he do, our friend Matt? He announces he's planning to talk to the Board and the press. I can't believe you haven't heard about this. It's been the news of the decade in the faculty lounge."

Kate stared at Eddie, dumbstruck. She had been too involved in her work to pay attention to the gossip in the faculty lounge and had, in fact, worked straight through lunch for the past two days. The bilingual research papers were turning out to be more challenging than she had anticipated, but she had committed herself to this project and was determined to see it through.

"Come on over to Shorty's. Matt's holding court there right now. Should be quite an event."

Kate shuddered to think of the ordeal her friend had in front of him, but his stubbornness would carry him through like a powerful launch cutting across a stormy sea. She rushed to gather her things and join the group at Shorty's.

The crowd had gathered, as Eddie had predicted, around a beat-up wooden table in the back room, where Matt sat with his feet up. His relaxed composure was clear evidence that he planned to win this battle; there was no way he was going to let the administration beat him.

Several teachers were leaning across the table toward Matt, almost surrounding him in their effort to be involved in his fight. Two teachers were talking at once, each offering 'the perfect approach' to take with the Board. Matt was trying to listen to both of them and the effect was like someone watching a ping-pong game played three inches in front of his eyes. Harry Carp was going through a list of points that Matt shouldn't forget to use in this argument.

After searching the group for someone remotely approachable, that is, someone who wouldn't hurl unjustified and unsolicited opinions at her before she'd even sat down, she spotted Mary Sinclair sitting alone, several tables away from the loud group. Mary smiled cordially, and Kate seized the opportunity to find out what she could about what Matt was up against.

An embarrassed silence ensued as each woman assessed the situation which had, only a few months earlier, been the cause of the rift between them.

Less concerned about keeping face than Kate was, Mary avoided the difficult subject and focused on an easier one. "He's called the two local papers already and I think there are some reporters on their way over right now."

"No!" Kate was shocked, yet thrilled that Matt could have orchestrated this situation to his advantage so masterfully- and so quickly! She craned her neck to make sure he was not drinking anything other than the glass of orange juice he usually settled for, but he was blocked by six or seven people crowding around his table. She hoped he was being sensible.

"You know how I feel about this, Kate," Mary said, preempting anything Kate might have said. "The main thing is that it's getting out in the open and the authorities will have to make a decision either way. Personally, I would have Matt take a leave of absence until he is definitely fit to teach again. But it's not up to me." She shrugged, not so much in defeat as in conscious detachment.

"Oh, my God!" Kate jumped up when she saw the newspaper reporters enter the bar. "They've got all those cameras, Mary. I can't believe this."

When the accident had first happened, six months earlier, coverage had been minimal because the school had suppressed most of the story. At that time, Matt had not been interested in "justice" and had refrained from the acrimonious actions suggested by Sam and a few others. But, after the most recent run-in with Alan Coon, where the principal had insulted his intelligence by reading an article on epilepsy aloud, Matt was ready to defend his rights.

A reporter with large, mournful cow eyes approached Matt and put a fat hand on his shoulder. "Mr. Reynolds," he drawled, "I would like you to tell this story to me like you're telling it to the entire population of Phoenix and Scottsdale. Because that's who's going to hear about it." Beside the empty beer bottle on the table, the reporter placed a small tape recorder whose red light was already beckoning to the storyteller in Matt.

"Wait!" the reporter said, waving his arm through the air as though to erase anything being said. "Caroline! Get over here and take a picture of Mr. Reynolds." He summoned the young female photographer with a snap of his fingers.

"Yes, Mr. Martin," the woman sighed, pushing past the onlookers to get to the table.

Matt eyed the obnoxious reporter narrowly, but warmed immediately to Caroline, who was busy trying to create a decent set out of the table and chairs. Someone moved the beer bottles out of the way ("don't want people to get the wrong idea, you know") and Caroline took three or four shots. On Matt's insistence, she took two pictures of Matt with some of the other teachers. Kate declined his wave to join them for a group photograph.

Finally, before Matt would let Mr. Martin get on with his story, Matt thrust the camera into his plump hands and demanded he photograph Caroline and him, arms raised in triumph.

"That one is not going to be seen by anyone," Caroline threatened, but with a hint of a smile playing at her lips.

"Okay, okay," said the reporter, impatiently. "We've got a story to tell here." He leered at Matt. "Give it all you've got."

And Matt gave it all he had, and then some. Shorty came over with some complimentary beers and sat down on a stool nearby to hear the story firsthand.

As Matt talked, the reporter bobbed his head up and down like a decoy on a duck pond, fishing for more details. He spluttered a few congratulatory remarks, smacked his lips several times, then snapped off the recorder.

"Beautiful. Beautiful. It makes my heart bleed."

I can't believe that, Kate thought to herself. She edged her way past a few other sycophants till she was directly across the table from Matt.

"Do you want a ride maybe, or…" her eyes flitted over to where Caroline was packing up her cameras.

"Yes, let's go." He bade his "fans" goodbye, shook Caroline's hand a bit too formally, then practically leapt out the door of the bar into the desert heat.

"And what was that innuendo back there?" he nudged Kate in the ribs as she started the car.

"Nothing. It's just that you're the biggest flirt I've ever seen in my life. Didn't you want her phone number?" (said with more than a touch of sarcasm).

"Hey," said Matt, squinting his eyes and snapping his fingers like a jaded movie star. "She knows where to find me."

"You're impossible!" she laughed. "Lovable, but impossible, all the same."

There it was, like a flash. The joy and the pain of wanting her, not for a brief instant, but forever. He breathed deeply through his nose and wouldn't look at her until he was sure it wouldn't show.

When Matt reached his office at the back of the gymnasium the next day, he could see a large sheet of newsprint practically covering the door. Oh no, he thought. But before he could get close enough to read it, a dozen students were pulling at his arm and slapping him on the back.

"Way to go, Mr. Reynolds!"

"Yeah, you tell 'em!"

Holding them off at arm's length, Matt scanned the article. It was amazingly accurate for newspaper reporting, he thought. The fat slob had actually heard what he had to say about the accident and the moral dilemma regarding his work with the kids.

"Now, listen," he said in a serious voice which silenced the students immediately. "Thank you for the support, but I will remind you that I'm just trying to do my job, which is to get you trained and ready for high school athletics. Now, don't forget that you have a job to do, too. And that is to try your hardest. *Don't* get distracted."

The hour that followed was one of the most tiring gym classes the students had ever experienced. Matt pushed them to their limits, stretching their wills along with their aching young legs. When the bell rang, he gave them a quick nod and slipped out the door.

"Very nice, Matt." Alan Coon's hunched stature blocked him from continuing down the hall. "That was a very tactless thing to do." The principal stood with his hands on his hips and his bottom lip jutting out.

Matt regarded him with a steely gaze. "I did not do it to insult you, Alan. It was something I had to do, and, to be fair, I think I could have said a lot more."

The two stood facing each other in a deadlock of strong wills, which Matt finally broke by announcing that he had an appointment. But Coon would not let him pass.

"We made a deal, Matt. The Board of Ed still needs to decide if you are fit to be working or not."

"We did not make any deal." Matt's eyes were slits boring a hole in the principal's pasty face. "And as far as I'm concerned, they've decided by default. They haven't come up with enough to keep me away, so I'm back. Now, if you'll *excuse* me..." He had to shove Coon's arm to get past him and he noted with amusement how flabby it was. He could recommend some exercises to improve the muscle tone, if he felt like being mean. But, for now, his primary concern was getting to Dr. Anderson's on time so he could settle this medication issue once and for all.

The doctors' offices were always hot and stuffy, Matt noted with disgust, wishing he were anywhere else. He rolled up his already-short sleeves and Kate made a face, mouthing the word "show-off" to him. He pulled the cuffed sleeves down slightly in an embarrassed attempt to hide his large biceps.

This was the first time that Kate had accompanied him to a doctor's appointment. The other times, she had dropped him off, then returned a half-hour later to collect him. It still bothered Matt tremendously that he had to rely on others to drive him everywhere. He hated the feeling of dependence that this caused, but the frustrating fact was that until he had two years completely free of seizures, or three years of only mild seizures in his sleep, he was not allowed to drive a vehicle of any kind.

Two years! He cursed inwardly. He could not even remember two months without a seizure. Luckily, none of the recent ones had been particularly massive, but he always tensed up when he felt the slightest bit strange.

Flipping through a three-month old magazine on nutrition, Kate looked serene. It had been her idea to be present at this appointment and although Matt had mixed feelings about her hearing the details that they would inevitably discuss, he wanted her there for moral support.

"Hey, come on, Matt. She's waving to you." He had not been concentrating on anything but Kate's lean brown leg showing beneath a gauzy floral skirt.

After an initial protest, the doctor agreed to let Kate remain in the office during the consultation, "as long as it's all right with Matt."

"I don't feel like the medication is doing anything to control my seizures and I'd like to stop taking it." Jumping right in, Matt had not even given Dr. Anderson the chance to open her file.

She shook her head. "We'll talk about this, but don't do anything stupid like stopping abruptly. That could set off all kinds of reactions in your brain." She pulled down a heavy tome from a shelf and opened it to a page that was marked with a postcard. Obviously, she and Matt had referred to this page before.

"Yes, yes, I know," Matt sighed, preempting Dr. Anderson's next comment. "We have several choices of medication, depending on the types of seizures I've been having. We've already changed medications twice and the dosages countless times. I'm tired of it!"

Kate had never seen Matt this worked up. She glanced surreptitiously at Dr. Anderson, who was remarkably composed as she touched her fingertips together lightly. Maybe they had had this conversation before, too.

"Kate will tell you how moody the drugs can make me sometimes." He pointed at her, a cue to turn on that moral support she had promised.

Moody. Yes, she would tend to agree with that. But hadn't Matt always been that way? It was so hard to remember anything from before the accident. "Well…" she stalled. "I've noticed that in the past few months Matt has been especially tired, whereas before he seemed to have unlimited energy. I don't know if that is a side-effect of the drug."

"We've discussed that," said the doctor in a clipped, peremptory tone that did not invite any further comment. Kate stiffened, feeling snubbed. The nerve, dismissing Matt's fatigue like that. "I've got you signed up for some physiotherapy, Matt." Her voice had softened measurably. She handed him a sheet of paper. "That's the schedule. It shouldn't interfere with your work at Ramon."

So simple, she made it sound. "Excuse me, but what is the physiotherapy *for*, exactly?" Kate was genuinely curious.

"An all-over treatment to improve circulation and relieve the muscles that have been over-worked during Matt's attacks."

Matt got up suddenly and crossed the room to look out the window. In the parking lot, two children were chasing each other, while a third looked on, yelling encouragement. He smiled at the way the children could turn any location into a playground, even the parking lot of a doctor's office. He whirled to face Dr. Anderson.

"I have important work to do, Carol." (*Carol? Carol?!!!* Leave it to Matt to get on a first-name basis with his doctor).

"I know you do," said Dr. Anderson. "Do what I'm suggesting and you may be in much better shape to do that work."

"I *may*. I *may*. Do you know we've been talking like this for nine months? And nothing's changed. I'm still having just as many fits. I'll do the physio, but I want to go off the damn medication, all right?" He silenced her with a piercing stare.

She nodded knowingly, and Kate found herself nodding, too, like someone under a spell. Why did he want her here, again? Shit! What was it she was supposed to be doing? Providing moral support. But now they were leaving, Matt promising to show up for the first session in the whirlpool that Wednesday, and Carol Anderson promising to look into the issue of the medication again.

Chapter 19

The campfire crackled and hissed as Helen threw a semi-damp branch on top of the smoldering ones. It cast a jagged shadow across her face as she gave Kate a cat-like smile and inched closer to the fire's warmth.

Going camping at the lake was an event Matt and Sam had been trying to organize for the past two months and now, as the summer was winding slowly to a close, it had finally become a reality.

"Come over here, Kate. It feels wonderful." Helen beckoned to her friend, indicating a flat area next to her. She was especially thrilled to have been invited along, since she had grown closer to Kate over the summer and had a taste of the camaraderie that existed among Kate, Matt and Sam.

"Mmm," Kate conceded as she sat down on the ground. "This has been rather a perfect day, hasn't it, Helen?"

"Oh, but of course. We wouldn't have it any other way." She made a moue with her lips that sent Kate into hysterics.

"What in the world is that, your impression of Navajo with a touch of old English lady at a tea party?" Kate shrieked with laughter, and Helen followed suit.

"What are we missing?" Sam shouted as he and Matt poked their heads out of one of the tents.

"Girl talk!" Helen and Kate responded in unison, which brought on further fits of laughter.

Matt shook his head in mock disgust and he and Sam disappeared behind the tent flap again.

When the flap closed, Helen leaned closer to Kate and whispered, "I could just eat that man alive." Kate raised an eyebrow. "Oh, I don't think I'd ever, well, you know, I mean, we did have our chance in college."

So, nothing had happened. Why did Kate feel such a sense of smug satisfaction at hearing that? She was just about to ask Helen what kinds of things they *had* done together when Helen beat her to it:

"Have you and Matt ever…uh..have you ever done it?"

"No!" A bit too emphatically. "We're just friends."

"But you'd like to, wouldn't you?" Nudge in the ribs.

"Helen!" She didn't know what to say. Helen was looking at her expectantly. "He's very attractive, of course," she concurred.

"Very. What about my brother?" She changed the subject so adroitly that Kate was caught off guard.

"Sam and I are just friends."

"Just friends, just friends. I wasn't going to tell you this, but Sam was pretty hot for you when he first met you. He let it slip when he was talking with me and my mom."

Kate let that sink in. She could not believe he had spoken about his feelings with his sister and mother. She suddenly felt embarrassed and tried to think back to her last visit to the reservation, the day of the sandpainting. Had Mrs. Littlefoot looked at her any differently? She felt she owed Helen an explanation. "We've talked about it, but I really don't think we feel that way about each other."

They spent the next ten minutes arguing about whether or

not Kate loved Sam or Sam loved Kate, or in fact, if Kate loved Matt or maybe Matt loved Kate.

"I think perhaps it's Matt and Sam who love each other. What are they doing in that tent, anyway? Hey, you guys, come on out of there!"

The men exited the tent and joined Kate and Helen by the fire.

"Cozy. Where's the rest of the wood?"

"We used it all, Sam. How much do you think I can carry, anyway?"

"All right, guys. Quit your bickering." Matt took charge, as usual. "Kate, let's go get some more wood for the fire."

"But it's dark."

"So, take the flashlight."

Yes, she supposed they could use some wood. She scrambled after him, pointing the flashlight beam at the dirt path that led toward the trees.

"What's that?" Matt asked in a choked whisper as he grabbed Kate's arm.

She screamed and dropped the armload of branches she had been holding.

Hearing his chuckling, she flew at him. "Matt! How could you do that to me?"

"Scared of the dark? The creatures in the night?" He made snake-like movements up and down her arm.

"Stop it," she laughed and swatted at his hands.

Then the hands slowed to a smooth stroking motion, which made Kate shudder. She could see Matt more clearly now, her eyes used to the shimmery moonlight. He took one step toward her and in an instant he held her in a strong embrace.

They stood completely still for a long moment, where Matt feared she might break away, as she had so many times before.

But Kate reached up to touch his face. She matched his intense look and drew him closer to kiss him. "I've been wanting you for over a year, do you realize that?" As she whispered in his ear, she could hardly believe it was she who was saying the words.

"Lie down here." His voice was sexy, and wafted toward her in rich tones.

"But..."

"Come on." Matt's strong arms guided her to the ground. Their bodies fell together and Kate savored the feel of his back and neck as she ran her hands all over him.

"Ow!" Kate rolled on top of Matt to avoid the branches and twigs poking her in the back.

"Mmm, Kate. I want you, too. But you knew that." He began to undress her.

"Wait." She hesitated. "Not here."

"Why not? It's quiet, romantic. Perfect."

"It's just that I've never done it outside before."

He held her face in his hands. "There's a first time for everything." He ran his tongue lightly down her neck as he pulled off the sweatshirt.

Feeling her body reach out for him, Kate imagined what it would feel like when they finally touched each other, as she had pictured countless times before. She did want him so much, it was a physical ache, and the closeness was almost too much to bear. She helped him remove his shirt and stroked the broad chest that now lay exposed in the moonlight.

They pressed against each other, first hard, then more gently. They explored each other's bodies with passion, curiosity, and then joy. *This is really making love*, Kate thought briefly as they matched the rhythm of their lovemaking with a wide-eyed, eager kiss. She had waited so long for this moment that she could not resist coming quickly to orgasm, wrapping her body around him as closely as she could.

Matt held Kate's hand tightly as he reached the height of ecstasy, breathing, "I love you, I love you" into her ear.

She closed her eyes to make the perfect moment linger even longer. Resting her head on his chest, she could feel the rise and fall of his breathing, faster than normal, and the heartbeat underneath as well.

Had he actually said he loved her, or had she imagined it? She wanted to ask him what he meant, but the moment was so still and peaceful that she did not dare break the silence.

The hoot of an owl brought Kate to full awareness. How long had they been gone? Surely Sam and Helen would be wondering what had happened. She rose jerkily on one elbow and tried to peer in the darkness toward the campsite.

"Relax," Matt crooned, pulling on her elbow which made her lose her balance. "They'll figure it out." He kissed her softly on the lips. "Believe me. I don't think either of them will be very surprised."

That was probably true. But how would Helen feel now that Kate had actually done it with her old flame? She thought back to their conversation by the fire. Helen had just about pushed her into Matt's arms, implying that there was something intimate between them. And now there was! Matt pointed to the patch of sky directly overhead. "You see that bright light there, like a star? I think that's Venus. Not bad for our guiding light, huh?" He gazed at her fondly.

This was so strange. All of a sudden, it was different between them, as though someone had spun them around very quickly, leaving them disoriented, looking out at a new horizon. An entire year had passed, complete with ardent talks about finding the "ideal mate", but still Kate had not seriously entertained the possibility of being with Matt on anything other than a platonic level. His tone now was that of a lover, having appeared instantly like a sun over their new horizon.

Stop analyzing and just enjoy, she reminded herself a bit viciously, for she had lapsed into an old way of thinking, one that did not let the moment just *be*, without prejudice and without *thinking* about it.

"We could stay out here, you know," Matt said as he and Kate walked slowly back toward the campsite, hand in hand. Each carried a bundle of branches in his free hand.

"What, sleep outside?"

"Sure, why not? It's much more invigorating than being inside a tent. I've done it lots of times." Seeing her look of dismay, he added, "But never with a woman, and certainly not with a beautiful one like you."

She jabbed him in the ribs. Charmer! She had to admit, it was wonderful to be on the receiving end for once, after watching Matt charm so many other women, seemingly unintentionally, always wholeheartedly. Despite the surge of joy she felt, she still dropped Matt's hand as they neared the clearing where Sam and Helen were sitting by the fire. Not ready to come out in the open yet.

Helen was laughing and slapping Sam on the back as they approached; Kate and Matt could sense immediately that the two had shared some valuable time together while they were gone.

"Nice couple of twigs," Helen said with a smirk. "I can see what took so long."

Giving her an uncomprehending shrug, Kate busied herself with the branches. As she bent over the fire, she was glad no one could see the burning red of her cheeks.

As she and Helen attempted to make coffee a few minutes later, Helen explained that she and Sam had finally had a much-needed discussion about why they had grown apart over the past few years. Kate was thrilled for both of her friends, and almost convinced herself that that was the impetus behind leaving them alone for so long. But it did not take much prodding on Helen's part for Kate to blurt out that she and Matt had been intimate in the woods, and that it had been divine. They felt at peace, just then, as though nothing could touch the perfect happiness that each had experienced in the past hour.

The group roasted marshmallows, to Kate's horror ("Oh, well, I'll go back to health food tomorrow" as she stuffed another golden marshmallow into her mouth). Then Helen went off to sleep in the tent that was meant for her and Kate.

"So," Sam grinned. "When's the wedding?"

"You've missed it." Matt's response was instantaneous and delivered with a perfectly straight face. "What do you think we were doing in the woods, anyway?"

"You don't want me to say."

Kate was mortified. "Guys! Could you please lay off?" This brought further cackles that were met with friendly shoves.

"All right." Sam stretched. "I'm going to bed, or rather, to sleeping bag." He looked at Matt expectantly.

"I'll join you in a little while, buddy. We'll just make sure the fire's okay."

"Sure, whatever you say. Have fun." Exaggerated wink and a wave, then Sam went into the men's tent.

Then there was an enchanted silence, broken only by the crackling logs in the fire and the hoot of an owl in a nearby tree. Matt felt Kate's eyes upon him and he turned to look at her.

She combed his hair with one of the smaller twigs. "Before I forget, I've been meaning to thank you for your help on the bilingual program. It was a great success and I think we've made some important strides in this area." Kate had received a letter from Alan Coon the day before which commended her for her progress in bilingual education. Apparently, the parents of the participating students were particularly pleased. Kate was both shocked and pleased to receive such a letter from the principal who, she knew, had never been a great proponent of bilingualism. But now it had the attention of the board and the public at large.

Unfortunately, there was no mention of Matt's work, despite the fact that Kate's program was based on his original concept. She felt guilty to be taking all the credit when he had done so much to get her started. He had even practiced a few Spanish phrases with her to make the program run more smoothly. No end to his talents, she had concluded.

Now, he reached over and touched her hair so that they were attached by their fingertips and locks of hair like two primitive beings.

"I'd like to make more progress with the Mexican students next year," he said pensively. "I feel like I was distracted by a hundred and one things this past year."

"Distracted! You had to overcome some major challenges, I would say. Yeah, and you came out a hero, didn't you?" Matt had won the battle with the administration and had finished out the year, sending more students to compete in the county-wide tests than in any previous year.

Matt looked bashful, a look that was very becoming on his face, with a long piece of hair resting on his cheek. Kate was glad his hair seemed to have stopped falling out since he had reduced the medication. She brushed the hair away lovingly.

"My hero," she breathed, and they fell into a tender kiss and embrace. She stroked his arms thoughtfully, running her fingertips over the muscles she had seen so many times, yet never touched. She felt so lucky, as though someone had finally deemed it all right for them to be together.

A sip from his wine glass and the taste of Matt's mouth was all red wine. She opened her eyes for a brief second to let him pour some into her mouth. He placed his moist lips on hers and let the warm fluid fuse them together.

I must feel you again, Kate felt suddenly, and slid on top of him again. She was so hungry for him this time; although she felt him hard and ready for her, she wanted to make it last much, much longer.

Deftly slipping her top off, Matt held the small of her back and climbed on top. "I'm not too heavy for you, am I?" he whispered with a concerned look in his eyes. But he was keeping most of his weight off her with his powerful arms supporting him on the ground.

A small moan escaped Kate's lips as she felt him enter her again. Slightly sore from contact less than an hour ago, each movement was very intense and felt throughout her bloodstream. She let her conscious mind take over long enough to remind her not to make too much noise, then let herself go again. She felt the heat from Matt's body as she tried to pull him even closer.

His chest, now bare, clung to her breasts as they rose and fell together in a slow, rhythmic pattern. She wanted him closer, faster, harder, but he kept her on the brink for so long. Finally, he cupped her lower back with his palm and pulled her to him swiftly and tightly.

It was all she could do not to scream with pleasure as she felt herself climax and shudder over and over, with Matt still rock-hard inside her.

As the after-shocks rippled slowly away, Kate opened her eyes, which she had been squeezing shut. She could not suppress her smile. The love she felt for him was complete, although it had been so for a long time. *They* had completed it and in doing so had created an even stronger bond than that which they had enjoyed over the past year.

"But it's your turn now," she promised in a sexy voice. "How do you want it, slow or fast?" She wanted to return his powerful lovemaking, wanted to make him feel as good as she did now.

He said a surprising thing. "I don't actually want to come right now. There is so much power in it that would be wasted if I did. I just want to continue holding you and making you feel good."

His words caressed her like silk. As if on demand, she arched her back and clung to him very tightly as another orgasm shook her body. "Stop...stop," she laughed, trying half-heartedly to gain control. "What are you doing to me?" She felt they would melt together permanently if she experienced that again.

When Matt's eyes met hers, they sparkled in the moonlight.

"Don't you want one?" she prompted, willing to do anything for him.

"No, really, Kate," he smiled. "It's a proven fact that if a man can control the number of times he ejaculates, he will increase his power in many ways. The semen has so much power in it." He saw that she was disbelieving. "It's part of an Eastern philosophy." The principle was Taoist, he said, and he would lend her an excellent book which would explain it all.

She did laugh out loud at this, at their inability to keep their intellectual curiosity at bay. "What about me?" she queried, giving him a flirtatious smile. "Do I lose more power with each one?"

"*Au contraire,*" he whispered and, still rolling gently inside her, proceeded to prove it to her. "I do love you, Kate," he said earnestly, just as she reached the crest of the wave.

She gasped as loudly as she dared and collapsed, panting, in a heap. "Please, no more," she said, reluctantly pushing him off her. *That was incredible*, she told him with her eyes.

You deserved it, he replied silently. And his palms rested on her slightly damp body until they were both ready to get up.

"Well," Kate exclaimed with a hearty laugh. "I hope Sam and Helen are sound sleepers." She looked across the blackness at the tents.

They nearly spent the night sleeping outside, as Matt had suggested, but after contemplating the repercussions this might bring about, Kate declined and left Matt with a passionate good night kiss. "I'll take a raincheck. Sleep well."

The men cooked breakfast the next morning, to the encouragement of Helen and Kate who practically ate the eggs straight out of the pan.

"I don't know why everything tastes better outside," Helen said with her mouth full, "but who cares? This is unbelievable. Would you be my live-in cooks? I'll pay."

Sam scratched his head as though he were considering her offer, but Matt shook his head emphatically. "Sorry, Helen, but I couldn't bear to see you become a fat squaw. It would break my heart." He pinched her thigh through her jeans.

Kate's heart felt hollow for a second, observing this playfulness, but then she remembered that they had known each other years ago.

"Actually," Helen resumed, without missing a beat, "have

you guys ever considered moving in together? You know, rent out the other places and live like 'three's company'? You see so much of each other and it seems sad that you're all in your own individual apartments, like hermits." She also envied them sometimes, which she didn't say. Her own living arrangement on the reservation was far from private.

"Maybe," Sam nodded, and that was it.

Kate had never told either of them that she had almost asked Matt if he wanted to live with her to alleviate his fears about being alone with the epilepsy. It had not come up recently, but now that they were lovers...

There was no further mention of it as the group organized themselves to return home.

No sooner had Kate turned on the lights in the apartment when she heard Matt's distinctive knock on the door.

"So you're not sick of me yet?" she joked, but her voice trailed off when she saw his face. "What's happened?"

He handed her a folded piece of paper which showed the telltale signs of having been crumpled into a ball and then smoothed out again.

She read quickly and her eyes widened in horror. "No. It can't be true."

But it was true. Alan Coon had sent Matt an official letter to inform him that his contract would not be renewed for the following school year. The reason, the letter stated, was clear: his medical condition, as attested to by highly respected members of the medical profession, left him unfit to conduct physical education classes where a seizure could potentially cause harm to himself or the students. This was the conclusion of the investigation which had taken four months to complete.

"Can you contest it?" Kate asked in a small voice, not feeling overly optimistic even as she said it.

He shrugged. "I thought they were pleased with the physiotherapy and the fact that I haven't had an attack in over three months, not counting the brief absence I experienced that time watching television."

He looked so forlorn that she wanted to cradle him in her arms and comfort him, but she was worried about looking like she was taking pity on him. In the end, she gave him a friendly hug and tried to be nonchalant. "You'll beat this, you'll see. Just hang in there and don't forget I'm on your side."

Instead of the hug she was expecting in return, Matt gave her a brief nod and took back the dreadful letter. "I'll see you tomorrow," he mumbled and left quietly.

She remained standing in the center of the room for quite some time after he left, too stunned to move. This was terrible, no doubt. But they would find a way out of it. Things work out, they always do. Matt himself had taught her that.

Chapter 20

The bell was particularly jarring this afternoon, Kate noticed as she rubbed the back of her neck. A rare headache had been plaguing her most of the afternoon, intensifying instead of diminishing after the aspirin that Mary had kindly given her. Maybe she should have taken both of them. Ow! Damn. Well, at least the day was over.

Kate had been saddled with four extra large classes this year, students spilling into the aisles, seated on chairs borrowed from the two adjacent classrooms and instigating each other to more distraction than usual. It was challenging to keep their attention focused on Shakespeare, but Kate drew on the inner calm that she had developed through her own infrequent meditation, and this seemed to help.

"Screeeech!" The teenager jumped off his skateboard just before it crashed into the brick wall and used the thick rubber soles of his sneakers as brakes. Half-lost his balance, but only landed on one hand and jumped up with a flourish. Maybe it was intentional, some kind of trick.

"Uh, sorry Miss Bennett." He stuck his hands deep in the pockets of his Levi's and looked at the ground sheepishly.

Kate bit back a smile. "Peter, if you want to lose that skateboard, just keep riding it down the hall. Otherwise I suggest you take it outside where it belongs."

"Yeah." He practically ran toward the door, skateboard under one arm. *I sound like such an old hag*, Kate thought. Pathetic.

"I hope you told him off but good" Mary. Who else?

"Hi, Mary. Peter's okay. He's just bored, I think he has to wait around until four when his mom picks him up on her way home from work."

"He could be studying instead. Now, *there's* a radical idea."

What a hard woman, Kate thought, incredulous. She didn't understand what was behind the bitterness.

"Come on, Mary," she said suddenly. "Let's go over to Shorty's for a drink."

"Oh, I don't know."

"Come on, just a quick one." Do us both some good she figured.

Halfway through the second Bud Lite, Kate leaned back in the booth and picked at the label that was peeling off from the condensation.

"How are you doing Mary?"

The other teacher was surprised.

"I'm fine. Why do you ask?"

Kate shrugged.

"I just thought you were looking a little stressed and I hoped everything was all right, that's all." She patted Mary's arm to soften the implication that she was prying.

There was a long silence while both women sipped their beers; Kate was reluctant to speak again because she could tell Mary had something on her mind. Sure enough.

"My sister Angela just found out she has leukemia. I think it's pretty far along. I've gone to have my bone marrow tested, but it doesn't match."

She threw her head back, looked at the ceiling for the answer.

"God, Mary, I'm so sorry to hear that. It must be an awful shock. Where does she live?"

"In Los Angeles. Luckily it's not too far away. I'm driving out on Saturday."

More silence.

"The worst part is listening to her talking about death. She wants me to take care of my niece Stephanie, if it does happen. Oh, I can't bear to think about it." She choked on a sob as the tears started running down her cheeks uncontrollably.

"Oh, Mary."

Kate kept her hand on Mary's shoulder. After a minute, Mary took the napkins from under their beer bottles and blew her nose. It was so funny seeing her wipe her eyes with the tacky 'Go for the Gusto' cocktail napkins that Shorty had chosen that Kate laughed out loud.

She saw Mary's eyes widen and just pointed to the remaining napkins, hoping she would see the humor.

Mary smiled. "Yeah, thanks for listening, Kate. Jesus, what am I going to do if Angela doesn't make it ? I mean I don't know anything about taking care of a thirteen year old girl."

"Yes you do. What about all your experience at Ramon ? I'm certain you'll be able to handle what ever happens. Don't worry about *that*. But for now, the important thing is that you are there for Angela now."

Saying this made Kate think of Matt, with the small stab of guilt she usually felt doing things without him these days.

Since classes had started, Kate had tried to visit Matt several times a week and keep him up-to-date with news about her classes and everything going on at the school, but it was difficult to know if he appreciated the permanent reminders of how much he liked Ramon, and how much he missed it.

"Mary, I'm going to run now," Kate said. "But you know my telephone number. Give me a call anytime if you want to talk. I mean that."

"Thanks, Kate." The other teacher's eyes did not quite meet hers and Kate guessed that she had made her feel slightly self-conscious, considering their tenuous relationship in the past.

"Thank *you*, Mary, for sharing your problem with me. I feel honored."

It was not often, she reflected later, that you got so many extra chances to be a good person, a truly good person, and Kate was thankful that somewhere deep in her subconscious, she had seen fit to let bygones be bygones and concentrate on what mattered, which was being a good friend to Mary. Jesus, the anguish that Mary must be going through now, knowing her sister would not be around much longer. Not having any brothers or sisters made it difficult for her to feel exactly what Mary must have been feeling, but it must be similar to caring about a very good friend. She drove faster.

"Nothing much." This had become Matt's standard response to Kate's standard question about his activities.

She absentmindedly picked up a towel that lay sprawled across the carpet. "I see you've been to the pool again. Is that getting any better?"

He shrugged. "It's all right, I guess. The physiotherapist is impressed with my strength, but she never saw me a couple of years ago when I was in top form." His eyes glazed over as he reminisced wistfully.

This was getting so difficult. Kate did not understand why Matt wanted to withdraw from her, whom he had called his "best friend". Every time she visited him these days, it seemed like pulling teeth to get him to talk about himself. He seemed perfectly content to let her go on about her classes or anything else in her life, but when it came time to open up about his own daily routine or anything that was personal, he was unwilling.

"I don't know what's with you, Matt, but you might want to snap out of it. Or don't, but stop taking it out on me." She was surprised to find the tears spring to her eyes.

Although it was not intentional, her tears succeeded in getting through to him and he was at her side within seconds. "Hey. Don't cry. I'm sorry. I'm sorry I've been such a recluse and such a damn pathetic, self-pitying..." he searched for another word. Unable to find one, he hugged her tightly instead. It was such a normal act for Matt to put his own concerns to one side the minute he sensed someone else needed his help.

As they cleaned up his apartment, which he had neglected over the last few weeks out of depression, Matt remarked how empty he felt without his work. He honestly felt like he could have kept teaching, possibly with a few modifications to the structure, but the decision had been final. To take any kind of legal action was bound to drag on for months, with no guarantee that the end result would be in his favor.

Instead of fighting in the usual Matt Reynolds style, he had become apathetic and depressed. He had never really seen any problem before as completely insurmountable. Therefore, he had no idea how to act and didn't do anything.

"I know something you'll like," he said, somewhat more brightly. "I've had all this time to work on my guitar and I think it's really improved. Tell me what you think." He sat on the edge of an armchair, resting the guitar on his knee.

Seeing him like that and hearing the mellow country-western music emanate from the instrument and his lips made

Kate recall the first time they met, at the annual Sunny Vista event. She closed her eyes for a moment, letting the music wash over her. All at once, the other, more complicated, emotions engendered on that day were vivid and all-encompassing. She had forgotten what a turmoil that instant infatuation with Matt had caused.

"'*Desperado*,'" he began the all-too-familiar Eagles song. "'*Why don't you come to your senses...*'"

"Hey! Hey! Do you mind? You're not going to drag *me* down into a quagmire of self-pity."

He looked at her, more puzzled than offended. "Okay, okay." Brief pause. "So, do you think my playing's improved at all, with all the practice I've been getting?" Little boy look that defied her to say no.

She laughed heartily. "You'll never change. Always fishing for compliments. Yes, actually, I think you do sound quite a bit better. That's really great." She meant it.

The guitar now rested against a pile of clothes which they had gathered, creating a bizarre still-life to depict what his life had become. He surveyed the scene carefully. "What I'd really like to do is write a few more of my own songs. I just haven't felt up to composing lately."

His own songs. Kate had never heard any of these songs, although Matt had alluded to them a couple of times. She debated whether or not to ask him. But things had been utterly and irreparably (?) different since they had returned from the camping trip to find Alan Coon's letter. It was as though the veil that had been so carefully and lovingly lifted over the course of the weekend had slammed down again in one fell swoop, turning into granite as it did so. She wanted so much for them to be able to recapture the mood of the camping trip, which, for her at least, had been heaven.

Luckily, they had remained good friends, as close as they had ever been, but that romantic element was no longer accessible. As quickly as she had allowed herself to feel something stronger for this man, she made excuses for the love they had curtailed themselves. Just a few days before the camping trip, when there were signs of something more, Kate had actually contemplated what it would be like to be married to Matt. Marriage was a very scary thought, after what she had been through with Mitch, but Matt was so unlike Mitch in every way that she could hardly even classify the two in the same way.

"How about pizza?" she asked. "You don't really feel like cooking anything, do you? I certainly don't."

"Fine, but let me order. They always make this special kind for me." Matt was in his element again, chatting with the pizza maker about the latter's family and recent trip to Italy. *He really takes a genuine interest*, she realized. *He's not just being polite.* She snickered as Matt tried a few Italian phrases on the telephone, then tried them again, obviously having been corrected by the person at the other end.

When he hung up the telephone, she asked him how he managed to get along so well with so many different kinds of people.

"I don't know. I've never really thought about it before." He scratched his head. "I guess I've always felt that everyone has something interesting to offer. Don't people just amaze you, with all of their stories and idiosyncrasies? I don't think I've ever been bored talking with someone." He mulled this last statement over as though hearing it for the first time.

"Don't people get on your nerves sometimes? How about Alan Coon? You can't tell me that you really have any good feelings about him after what he's done to you?" She gave him a challenging look.

"Well, I do think Cooney is interesting as a psychological study. Of course, he's really made me angry, but at the same time, I can see his point of view. He feels strongly about my not putting the kids in danger. I don't think he had it in for me personally. Oh, that reminds me, the insurance claim has finally been settled, and the school is going to pay for all those hospital bills I've been ignoring."

"That is good news. But I still think if I were you, I would not give Alan Coon the time of day. I don't think he's worth it. Do you know, he gave me so many students in my ninth grade literature class that it's a fire hazard? He doesn't care. He doesn't see my point of view."

"But what can he really do? The students needs to take the class. He doesn't have the budget for any more staff. Maybe you could use a different classroom for that particular class. I know it would be a hassle, but if you're breaking the fire code now…"

"Maybe." It was a good idea. "But it still infuriates me that he has not helped me deal with this situation up to now. Oh, I don't wish to lose my appetite talking about that man now, do you mind?" She flung her hand out, as though erasing all traces of Alan Coon.

The pizza arrived before they could embark on any other controversial subjects. Matt had ordered a large, which, to Kate looked extra-large, and he was halfway through his second piece while she was still burning the roof of her mouth with her first.

Matt's dog, Yellowstone, padded up to them shyly, smelling the spicy aroma but not wanting to beg. Matt gave Yellowstone a long string of cheese that was clinging to the box; he and Kate laughed as the dog snapped his mouth open and shut several times in an effort to get the stringy cheese off his chin. Matt finally plucked it off himself and shoved it into the dog's drooling mouth.

Kate was disgusted. "And now you're going to continue eating with your hands all full of dog saliva?"

He nodded happily. "He's very clean, you know. Probably has fewer germs than you and I do." He leaned towards Kate, threatening to kiss her on the lips.

Even as she backed away in mock horror, she noticed how much she missed touching Matt and kissing him. It had been six weeks since classes started and this was the first time they had teased each other like old times. She put her piece of pizza down and kissed him on the lips before he could say anything. "You see, I'm not scared of a few germs."

The kiss was long and hard, smoothing over the rift created in the past six weeks. Kate finally broke away, breathless. "Wow, what on earth was that?" She pushed her plate to one side and rubbed up against him. "Come on, we can always heat the pizza up later."

Matt held her a few inches away. He looked upset as he said, "I don't know, Kate. I haven't been feeling right these past few days. I'm pretty sure I had a major seizure in my sleep last night."

"Why didn't you tell me?" She was outraged. "Are you still trying to be the martyr and deal with this on your own? Because if that's the way you want it, I'll leave you alone to deal with it." Her voice broke and she looked away from him to regain her composure. "I care about you so much, Matt."

He nodded, stroking her hair. "I know. And I care about you too, which is why I don't think we should be involved like that. I don't want you to be hurt any more than you have been already." So at least he acknowledged that.

"What about the medication?"

"I'm only on a small dosage now. It's better than before. I don't get as tired anymore."

She shook her head. "But the seizures have not stopped?"

"I don't know. Like I said, it happened in my sleep, most likely. When I woke up, I was still in bed, with the covers wrapped around me. I just felt like shit, that's all."

They sat in silence for a few minutes. Kate had never felt as helpless as she did at that moment. *Don't shut me out!* she wanted to scream. *Let me comfort you.* But Matt did not seem to want to be comforted.

She stroked his arm slowly; he did not push her away. "Matt," she began nervously, "you can't deny that there's something special between us. It's not the kind of feeling we should just toss aside, either." The shakiness had left her voice, replaced with a rich sense of confidence. She moved to kiss him again.

As gently as he could, Matt averted his face. "I'm sorry, Kate." His face was a picture of misery and he looked like he was fighting inner demons. "I'm just not in a position to love you the way you deserve to be loved. Believe me, Kate, this is killing me."

The quiet in the room was unbearable. Kate felt like she had heavy weights on her arms, holding her back from hugging him fiercely, the way she wanted to.

"Do you want me to leave now?" she asked quietly.

"Yes, I think so." There was nothing left to say. She went out the door quickly, blinded by the tears stinging her eyes.

Chapter 21

The telephone rang just as Kate had slammed the front door. She fumbled with the keys, cursing the lock, the phone and the caller.

"Oh, George! Good to hear your voice. She's in labor?!!! Oh, my God. How are you coping?" It was unbelievable that this day was finally here. Although several of Kate's friends had had babies over the past few years, they had not been close friends like Jackie. With Jackie's lively descriptions of every step of the pregnancy, Kate almost felt like she had gone through it herself. And now, any time now, the twins would be born. Kate, Sam, and Matt planned to visit George and Jackie next month for a long weekend, to catch up and celebrate the birth of the babies.

"I'll let Matt know. We're heading out for brunch now ourselves. He'll be thrilled. Give Jackie a big kiss for us. We'll see you in just a few weeks."

She practically flew out the door and across the courtyard to Matt's apartment. The phone call had made her even later and he was sure to be as hungry as she was by this time.

Ringing the doorbell for the third time, Kate wondered if Matt was out back practicing his karate or something. The door was locked; at least he had started to heed her warnings.

She wandered around the side of the building, but he was nowhere to be seen. She knocked on the sliding glass door and went in, one of Matt's own tricks.

"Matt? Are you home?" No answer. How could he have forgotten about their brunch date? He constantly told people that eating was one of his favorite hobbies. Maybe he was out on one of his morning walks in the mountains. She was wondering whether to wait there or go back to her apartment when Yellowstone whined from his spot on the floor. Kate had not even seen the dog until then.

"Where's Matt?" she asked, as though the animal could answer. The silence chilled her. No, don't be ridiculous. Stop overdramatizing everything.

Yellowstone whined again, more plaintively, and threw himself against the bathroom door. The bathroom?!

She took three steps toward the bathroom door and tried the handle. It was not locked, but a weight on the other side made it hard to open. Kate pushed Yellowstone away as gently as she could in her panic to open the door. "Matt?"

When the door finally swung open, the force was so great that Kate fell into the small room and practically landed on Matt, who was indeed lying on the floor. It took her a few seconds before she saw the blood all around his body. He must have fallen so hard! Seeing Matt on the floor reminded Kate so much of the seizure at her apartment and she suddenly felt weary and depressed. She leaned down to listen to Matt's breathing and it was at that moment that she saw the razor blade. The pool of blood was so large that she had not noticed before how it all stemmed from his wrists.

No!!! She could not hear any breathing at all. *No, Matt, you idiot! How could you do this?* She stared at the blood, willing it to enter Matt's bloodstream again and bring him back to life.

Then she fainted.

The Arizona desert always spread itself out like a vast brown carpet, the various shades of brown punctuated with the dusty green of the hardy cacti that thrived in the dry, intense heat. This was a desert in which Kate could lose herself, become part of the infinite brown and dusty green.

Sam's presence as he walked beside her was a comfort. The past two weeks had been fraught with pain and despair, as the finality of Matt's death impressed itself upon both of them with ever-increasing insistence. There had been all of the small details to deal with; Kate had taken it upon herself to handle as much as she could, so Mrs. Reynolds would not have to worry in her emotional state. The concentration on practical problems, such as Matt's personal effects, kept Kate's mind from dwelling on the inescapable hurt which still managed to course through her body each night anyway. She had taken a week off at Ramon, which Alan Coon did not dare to contest.

"Here, gorgeous." Sam handed her a tiny purple cactus flower.

"Sam. You didn't have to take it off the plant. You know how I feel about that."

He shook his head and smiled. "No, it's okay sometimes. The plant will produce more flowers. You deserve this one."

She took it reluctantly, then smiled. "Remember that trip to the reservation when we saw all the cacti in flower? That was when we first thought of doing the sand painting for him."

"When *you* first thought of it," he corrected her with a chuckle.

"Sam," she stopped in her tracks. "Do you think the sand painting did any good?"

"Of course it did. It's not a black and white kind of thing, where all of a sudden, everything's perfect. It worked in a more subtle way I think. You believed it worked at the time, didn't you? So, it did."

She nodded in agreement. "I have put the bear fetish on that shelf in my living room. Do you think I should give it back to Helen?"

"No. It was a gift. And now, it's Matt's gift to you. There are still powers in that little bear, if you believe in that."

She still felt a bit strange keeping the fetish. Matt had already given both of them so many gifts: his friendship and caring, his insights, his time. It was so hard to imagine life without him…She breathed deeply to allow the sob that was shaking her body to settle down. The purple flower in her hand seemed to take on a richer hue as it caught the solid sunlight of the desert afternoon. On a whim, Kate placed it in her hair. But her hands were so empty then, as if they were waiting for something to hold.

"He's affected my life like no one else. Rationally, I know that he is gone, but I still wish there were some way that I could turn the clock back and he would still be alive. Do you think that's silly?" Kate challenged Sam with an intensity in her eyes that he had never noticed before.

"It's not silly at all, Kate. No matter how 'rational' we think we are, when something like this happens, we can fall apart as easily as the next person." Sam's eyes were glassy as they threatened to spill over with his own tears. He wished he could let his emotions out more openly, like Kate did. He knew that if he demonstrated how he was feeling inside, he would be bawling now.

"I miss him too, you know. I miss him so much." He hoped she understood. "He's affected my life, too." Sam looked heavenward for a way to articulate how he was feeling. "It seems like he made me aware of what I already had inside," he said, finally, nodding as he spoke. "You know how people used to say that he and I had so much in common? Well, I used to feel embarrassed because I didn't think I had nearly as many good qualities as he had. But in his eyes I was okay. He always accepted people for what they are."

Yes, she knew that better than anyone. Matt had been such an inspiration to her as well, that it made her want to be the best she could be in everything. When she felt herself slipping into self-pity about his death, she reminded herself to be thankful for the time they had had together.

One tear made its way down Kate's cheek, despite her logical explanation. Instead of brushing it away, she let it paint a course on her skin and gradually evaporate in the hot afternoon sun.

"Sam, you would not believe how people are talking about Matt now. The ones who did not seem to show much sympathy during the past year are accusing him of committing some kind of sin. As if they have any right to judge him! And he can't even defend himself!" The tears were falling steadily now, in her indignation.

Sam stopped walking. "Then we have to defend him. You and I know what was really going on in his head."

Do we, she thought sadly. But, she could almost put herself into Matt's mindset, which was that of someone who had lost the battle he had entered so valiantly. No, that wasn't quite right. He hadn't lost. He only lost the vision and the energy to keep fighting. By taking his own life, he could still be a Samurai warrior and die "the honorable way", and not let the dreaded epilepsy claim his life in addition to everything else. She explained all this to Sam. "What do you think?"

"Yes, yes." He nodded vigorously. "The Samurai warrior wouldn't let his opponent get him first. Matt did the honorable thing. Never mind all the crap people will tell you about how it's not fair to those he left behind. He wasn't happy with the person he had become, and he couldn't bear to keep up the facade just for others. You know how many times he let it slip how tired he was."

"I'm tired, too, Sam. The whole ordeal has been so draining."

He touched the purple flower in her hair. "You'll be all right. So will I. We just have to think of the example Matt gave us and the difference he has made in our lives. We have every chance to make our lives into whatever we want. I for one feel like I have a new life ahead."

As they walked, the shadows grew longer, stretching into the distance. They forgot everything else except the soft sound of their footsteps in the dirt.

"I had a dream the other night." Kate wondered whether Sam would want to hear about the inane workings of her subconscious.

"Please go on," he prompted when she fell silent.

"You and I were walking along the highway, you know, the really flat part just coming out of Phoenix? Well, we walked and walked for what seemed like miles, and Matt was walking towards us from the other direction. You and Matt made some kind of secret sign to each other, like fraternity brothers or something." Sam smiled at this. "Then I started panicking, because although we were walking towards him and he was walking towards us, the distance kept getting bigger, he was getting farther and farther away. It was the strangest thing." She shook her head in disbelief. "And the worst part of it was that he was fading away, out of sight. I was running like mad, but there was no way I could get to him."

"What was I doing?" Sam was fascinated, hoped he had been running toward Matt also, in Kate's dream.

"You just kept making this strange sign with your hands." She tried to recreate the sign she had dreamt about, palms outstretched.

A shudder went through Sam and he suddenly felt cold all over. "Where did you see that?" he whispered harshly.

"In my dream." She bit her lip, uncomprehending.

"You must have seen it somewhere," he insisted, standing as still as a statue. He felt rooted to the ground, solid, omniscient.

"What's the matter?" The fear swept across Kate's body, but she waited for him to answer.

"That's part of a dance the Navajo do over someone who is dying."

Kate stifled a cry. "I don't know where I saw it, Sam. It was just a dream." Please don't get violent, she thought, which shocked her because she had never been afraid with Sam before.

He just nodded and drew some swirling lines in the dirt with a sharp rock. He recalled with interest the sign that Kate had made with her hands. Although the lessons in Navajo ritual had only begun a few weeks ago, Sam was learning rapidly. There was so much to learn, and it was so draining for some reason.

But this ritual was one that stood out in his mind because when the elders showed him, they had spoken in hushed whispers that lent even more mystery to the teaching. Grey Panther had said that when the spirit of the person was about to leave the body, the medicine man could help it begin its journey, pull it free from the material form that still held onto it.

What the hell did it mean, he asked himself furiously. He and Matt, both making the sign, then Sam making the sign by himself as Matt slipped from life to death? Yes, he knew the meaning: it was to encourage him to continue the lessons, to become a healer in spite of the gruelling work that lay ahead of him.

Next to him, Kate stood on her toes, trying to see farther into the distance as she shaded her eyes against the sun. He felt a pang then, for she had always been the one to support his ideas of getting back in touch with his heritage.

"Forgive me, Kate," he said in a low voice. "I didn't mean to shout like that. I don't know what got into me."

"It's okay," she smiled. "We're both going through so much emotionally. Don't worry about it." She paused. "It's unbelievable, though, isn't it? How it came to me in my dream like that."

Sam shook his head slowly. "Not so unbelievable." He watched an iguana slither out from under a squat cactus and make its way across their path.

"This desert," Kate spoke the words like an incantation. She was aware of the iguana crawling past her feet, but her eyes focused on the flat landscape. "It's so beautiful."

As he turned towards her, she could see that the wild fiery look had left his eyes. "He loved the desert so much," Sam said. His voice broke on the last word.

She gulped. "I know. He once promised me a slow dance out here, where there are no strobe lights. I'll always remember the time he came out with us to The Factor and he wouldn't go dancing because of the strobe lights. Come to think of it, I don't think he even wanted to be in the nightclub. I was so insensitive." She stomped her foot on the ground in anger.

When she didn't say any more, he asked her to explain. "Sorry," she said with a slight giggle. "Sorry, I got distracted. So, he asked me if we could go to the desert sometime and have a dance away from all the strobe lights and noise." She didn't need to add that it had never happened.

Sam slowly blew out a long breath. "There was always that touch of a poet in Matt. I don't think I'll ever be able to come and walk in the desert again without thinking of him." He took a pace towards Kate. He felt Matt's presence very strongly then, guiding him. Maybe he *had* had a part in the release of Matt's spirit. It was a comforting thought.

"If you want," Sam said slowly as he looked Kate in the eye, "we can dance a dance for Matt right now. If you think it's okay, of course." He looked almost shy as he held his hands outstretched to her.

"Yes," she nodded. It seemed fitting that they should dance in the desert and remember the person who had made such an impact on both of them. In the place that held so much meaning for all three of them. As they stepped slowly in time to the music of the wind, Kate felt her body relax and a spirit of survival take hold of her.

As Kate relaxed, Sam held onto her more tightly and the tears began to flow. He gasped for breath as he cried and cried, feeling everything come together for the first time. *Don't let go*, he pleaded silently to Kate, and whether it was because she read his mind or because she needed to hold onto him too, she remained in his arms for a long time.

The dance slowed almost imperceptibly until they were standing still.

Reluctant to let go of each other completely, they held hands as they began to walk back.

"I know what I forgot to tell you," Kate almost shouted,

her voice disappearing into the vast space. "Jackie and George have come up with names for the kids. Are you ready for this? Matt and Matilda. Do you believe it?"

Sam laughed and laughed, holding his sides. "Oh, God," he spluttered finally. "Those poor kids. Well, if they have any of his qualities, they're pretty lucky. I can't wait to see them next month." The trip to Denver would be even more meaningful now.

Kate smiled, thinking of Jackie and George and of Matt's namesakes. It seemed easier to cope with Matt's death when she realized the twins would be there from now on to remind them of him. Some joy to assuage their saddened hearts. Kate felt benevolent and expansive, at peace with herself for perhaps the first time.

A dark cloud had settled over the desert while they stood there, its heavy presence removing the rest of the landscape like a broom. There was a sudden clap of thunder and Kate quickly looked back at the car. But she knew it was too far to run and beat the rain that would pound down and drench them within seconds.

Afterword

Are you shocked and upset by the events in this book? Join the club! This book is based on a true story, and the hero did in fact take his own life. Unfortunately, in the real life version as in this fictionalized one, those of us who were close to the situation were paralyzed by fear and uncertainty, whereas it might have been more helpful to face our fear and never stop looking for ways to support our friend.

A Dance in the Desert aims to show how a talented young man could let a condition like epilepsy, and the social problems associated with it, demoralize him to such an extent that he would lose hope and take his own life. The main message I have for readers is that we all need to find within ourselves more love and support for people dealing with challenging situations. My heartfelt wish is that no one else with a health challenge like epilepsy should ever feel so helpless or desperate that he takes his own life.

From day one, half the profits from all my book sales have been donated to charities specializing in providing support for people with epilepsy and their families. This a major personal campaign and mission for me, not just to raise more money for the charities, but also to raise awareness of this very misunderstood condition, affecting up to one in twenty people. Most people with epilepsy live full and active lives and manage to control their seizures successfully with medication. There is, however, an increased risk of death due to accidents, suicide and other medical conditions. There are also cases where the death appears to be directly related to epilepsy itself, usually referred to as Sudden Unexpected Death in Epilepsy (SUDEP).

In 2003, I became an accredited volunteer with Epilepsy Action (the working name of the British Epilepsy Association, a registered charity in the UK). This charity supports over 22,000 members and operates an important telephone helpline that people can call to obtain information about epilepsy-related issues or speak to someone who understands the condition. If you would like to know more about the work of Epilepsy Action, please see the website www.epilepsyaction.org. The Epilepsy Foundation in the United States is another good resource—see www.epilepsyfoundation.org.

Thank you for buying this book, which will help the awareness and fundraising campaign. There are many other ways in which you can help, from spreading the message in this book, to getting involved in charities, but most importantly by offering your love and support to people you know with personal challenges. It does not matter what the *right* words or deeds might be, just follow your heart and help someone. It might save a life.

Mindy Gibbins-Klein
September 2004

About the Author

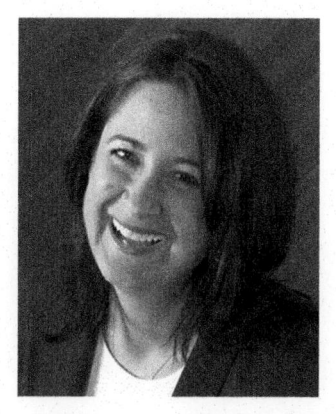

Mindy Gibbins-Klein experienced the pain of losing two close friends to epilepsy. She believes in the power of the human spirit and spiritual friendship. She has chosen to set the novel in Arizona, where she spent time working, and which has always been a very spiritual place for her. Since first publishing *A Dance in the Desert* in 2001, Mindy has written and edited three more books, and she founded The Book Midwife, a coaching and consultancy company dedicated to helping aspiring authors pursue their dream of getting into print. She also became an accredited volunteer with Epilepsy Action, the UK's largest epilepsy charity.

She currently resides in London, England with her husband and two children.